Come Alive!

FEEL FIT-LIVE LONGER

DON HAWLEY

Review and Herald Publishing Association
Washington, D.C. 20012

Copyright © 1975 by
Review and Herald Publishing Association
Library of Congress Catalog Card No. 75-21190

Editor: Raymond H. Woolsey
Cover: Mark English
Book Design: Alan Forquer

Printed in U.S.A.

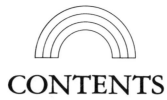

CONTENTS

To
Craig and Sheri

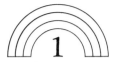

ZOMBIES
ARE FOR REAL

IN CERTAIN parts of the world superstitious people believe in frightening apparitions called zombies. These creatures are supposed to be the walking dead, who have somehow been reactivated through sorcery. Of course, educated people know better than to believe in such fantasies, but reasonable facsimiles of zombies are everywhere abroad in the land. You may know a few of them personally. In fact, you may even *be* one!

How do you know whether you qualify? It's easy to tell. Just consider these simple questions: Is the ringing of your alarm clock each morning the most unpleasant sound you can think of? Do you sit dazed on the edge of the bed for several minutes before summoning up enough strength to tackle showering and dressing? Does your stomach rebel at anything more than a slice of white toast and a cup of black coffee for breakfast? Does the morning rush-hour traffic deposit you at the office as tense as a tightly wound spring?

Does your already meager store of strength begin to fade about midmorning, and do you then down a cola drink for a quick "pick-me-up"? At noon do you try to recoup your reserves with a hamburger, French fries, and a malt? Is your personal midafternoon energy crisis so persistent that

the rest of the day finds you merely going through the mo-
tions of working? Do you eat a large evening meal, but
still find you've only sufficient strength to make it to your
favorite chair in front of the TV set? Do you doze through
the late show and then collapse into bed, wondering
whether there isn't something more to life?

If you answered Yes to most of the above questions,
you qualify: you are a practicing zombie. This doesn't
make you peculiar, of course, just one of the crowd.

Is there a design problem?

Why is it so many people feel dragged out, only half
alive? Is this a normal state of affairs? Something we just
have to learn to live with? Is the human body so poorly
designed we can't cope with the rigors of life?

Allow me to answer that last question first. There's
nothing wrong with the design of the human body. It's
the most complex and exquisitely fashioned mechanism
in the entire world. In fact, we have no right to take ourselves so much for granted.

An entire library of physiology books couldn't do
justice to the intricacies of the human body, but let's
ponder just a facet or two. First of all, whether you are
president, plumber, or poet, you started out as did everyone else, as a single cell. And that cell was so tiny as to be
invisible to the naked eye. Even so, the miracle of life was
well under way. By the time the doctor slapped your bottom and you responded with a lusty squall, you could
boast some 200 billion cells.[1]

And talk about gaining weight. During that same nine-
month period you increased your weight by a phenomenal
2 billion times! One scientist has estimated that "if a person continued to grow after birth at the same rate the
embryo grows inside the uterus, by the time the person
was an adult he would be as big as the world." [2]

But back to that original cell. Locked into that microscopic little bit of protoplasm was the entire you. Your

brown hair and brown eyes, your five-foot-seven-inch height, your pleasant singing voice, and even the way you walk. Then, in a still poorly understood manner, that one tiny cell produced more than 200 other highly specialized types of cells. One group developed into a rigid framework called a skeleton. Another group became muscle tissue so attached to the skeleton as to make movement possible. One group formed a small pouch, the stomach, to help process your food. And on and on. Fantastic!

One square centimeter of miracles

One more brief illustration will help to show how wonderfully complex you really are. Let's bypass the more glamorous organs, such as the heart and the brain, and consider something apparently uncomplicated—your skin. After all, this is only the wrapping for the human package. And we'll concentrate on only a very small portion at that; only one square centimeter on the back of your hand. That is a patch of skin about this big:

Now stand by for a surprise. The more than 3 million tiny cells that make up that little patch of skin are unbelievably specialized. Packed into that tiny area are:

 1 yard of blood vessels to provide nourishment
 4 yards of nerves to carry messages
 10 hairs
 2 sensors to detect cold
 12 sensors to detect heat
 15 sebaceous glands to keep the skin supple
 25 pressure organs for sensing touch
 100 sweat glands to carry off impurities
 200 nerve endings to record pain

I can almost hear someone saying, "Granted that my body is a complicated mechanism. But if it is so exquisitely designed, then how come it's out of whack so often?

How come I have a toothache on Monday morning, a dizzy spell on Wednesday afternoon, and a full-blown case of the flu by Saturday night?"

Yes, the world seems to be one vast storehouse of sickness and disease. To wish someone a "Good morning, how are you?" is to invite a long litany of assorted aches and pains. What's wrong with this human race? Don't we care about being well?

What people really want

A study was made recently to learn what people want out of life. What do you think topped the list of desires: world peace? financial gain? More than anything else, respondents listed good health. And as for fears, more than anything else, including the threat of atomic disaster, they feared ill health.[3]

Obviously, something is radically wrong. That which we most fear is almost constantly with us, and what we most desire seems to elude us. This is a tragic state of affairs. The purpose of this book is to help people avoid that which they most fear and to attain what they most desire.

We want to proclaim boldly that a state of illness, or even living with that "dragged out" feeling, is not normal. Average, perhaps, but not normal. The simple, basic health principles in this small volume, if incorporated into the daily life, will result in a vitality and sense of well-being you may never have experienced before. And it won't take ten years to feel the difference; benefits will be realized in weeks or months. Turn in your membership card to the zombie cult, and join those who truly live. Come alive—now!

---

[1] H. Shryock, M.D., *Your Amazing Body* (Nashville, Tenn.: Southern Publishing Association, 1971), p. 15.

[2] The *Miracle of Life* (Chicago, Ill.: American Medical Association, 1970), p. 4.

[3] *Health Insurance News* (New York, N.Y.: Health Insurance Institute, February, 1974), p. 1.

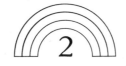

HIGH-LEVEL
WELLNESS

HEALTH IS tremendously important. People in the United States spend about $100 billion a year trying to restore and maintain it. This nation's health facilities employ more people than any other industry except construction. We took note earlier of the fact that health is what people desire more than anything else in the world. Health is a top priority item, all right—but have you ever tried to define it?

"That shouldn't be too difficult," you may be thinking. But just give it a try; you'll find it isn't easy. In fact, definitions of health have varied greatly through the years. Let's look at a few.

"You're healthy if you don't feel sick." This idea once satisfied most people, even though it isn't true. A person may feel perfectly well and still be harboring a dangerous or even fatal condition in his body.

"Health is distance from death." That's an interesting concept, isn't it? When it comes to death, we'd all like to keep our distance.

"Health is freedom from disease." Now that sounds like a simple statement of fact, doesn't it? But it presents only a very limited view of what health really is. We observe

many people around us who are not afflicted with any specific disease or infirmity, yet some of them obviously enjoy better health than others. Up to this point all of our definitions have actually been telling us what health is *not*. Let's move away from these narrow and constrictive viewpoints to something more positive.

Health is *"the state of being hale, or sound in body, mind or soul, especially freedom from physical disease or pain,"* according to Webster's New Collegiate Dictionary. A step in the right direction. C. L. Marshall in his book *Dynamics of Health and Disease* arrives at an interesting conclusion. "A person can be ill and well simultaneously. . . . Millions of Americans whose blood pressure is too high or whose blood sugar is abnormally elevated function without any difficulty whatever. . . . Health and disease are not opposites—both may coexist in the same person." [1]

A new approach to health

In 1947 the World Health Organization, established by the United Nations, put its prestige and influence behind a new approach to the understanding of health:

"Health is a state of complete physical, mental, and social well-being and not merely the absence of disease or infirmity." The word "complete" may make this definition seem rather Utopian, but at least it presents a positive and worthy goal.

Perhaps health may best be thought of in terms of degrees. Sometimes, even though you are not suffering from a specific illness, you feel worn out. You are listless, and nothing seems interesting or particularly worthwhile. It takes all the energy you can muster just to struggle through the day. Life hardly seems worth the living.

On the other hand, some days find you full of zip. Every cell in your body seems to be electrically charged. You plow through a heavy work load with very little fatigue, and it's great just to be alive. Right?

Now, what makes the difference? Using one of the narrow, restricted views of health, you were "well" on both occasions. But it is obvious that on some days you are "well-er" than on others. There are, then, degrees of health.

Any intelligent person who has a choice would surely opt for a life of dynamic buoyancy as opposed to a dragged-out, half existence. Well, we do have a choice. And the purpose of this book is to help you attain—and maintain— a state of *high-level wellness*.

People and frogs are different

In high school biology lab we spent considerable time cutting up frogs that had been preserved in formaldehyde. Such dissection experiments proved to be both interesting and informative. However, when it comes to people and treating their illnesses, subdivision into many medical specialties can have drawbacks.

Of course, we all appreciate the expertise demonstrated by the various specialists, and most of us have benefited from their skills. But often we feel a bit disjointed. It is as if the cardiologist appears to see us only as a heart, the ophthalmologist as a pair of eyes, the dermatologist as an envelope of skin, et cetera. Sometimes we feel like calling out, "Hey, I'm not just an anatomical jigsaw puzzle; I'm *me.*"

It is encouraging to hear that the "family physician" is making a comeback. I think he'll receive a warm welcome, although he will still seek the services of a specialist whenever indicated. While it's true that the human body encompasses a number of intricate systems, including the circulatory, the nervous, the digestive, the glandular, and others, we are more than ever aware that all these systems are interconnected and interdependent. And although the mental faculties are something above and beyond mere physical dimensions, we are beginning to realize that multifaceted man must be treated as a whole. He is body, soul, and spirit, and any meaningful health care must be directed to his entire being.

Caring for the whole man

The "whole man" concept of health broadens our horizons considerably. John LaPlace puts it this way:

"The contrast between the traditional and the contemporary concept of health is significant. The traditional notion that health is simply absence of disease or injury helped only in a simple sense. Sick or uncomfortable patients went to the doctor. He prescribed treatments which, if they worked, restored what was considered to be health. The removal of the complaint was all-important. It rarely occurred to the doctor to ask about the home life of the patient or about successes or failures in his social relationships. Such factors seemed relatively unimportant if a person suffered from severe indigestion or high blood pressure. It took time to realize that these factors did matter, and mattered a great deal.

"Today we understand that family pressures can contribute to high blood pressure, and that tension on the job can trigger indigestion. We have developed a more comprehensive and more workable definition of health." [2]

As vital as good health is, its attainment should not be our only interest. We are not advocating faddism or extremism. Health is not an end in itself, but a means of attaining to life's great purposes.

In the past we have tended to think of health almost solely on a *quantitative* basis. The "healthy" person was the one who avoided disease and outlived most of his friends and relatives. But even more imporant is the *quality* of life. Not merely how much life, but what kind of life. We'll discuss this in depth later on. For the time being, let's remind ourselves that good health is a positive, dynamic state of being. And we should not settle for anything less than high-level wellness.

---

[1] C. L. Marshall, *Dynamics of Health and Disease*, 1972.
[2] John LaPlace, *Health* (New York: Meredith Corporation, 1972), p. 2.

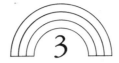

HOW TO
BURN YOUR CANDLE

IT WAS an exciting day in the life of a young medical student at the University of Prague. The year was 1925. Hans Selye had applied himself faithfully to his books on anatomy, physiology, and biochemistry, but now he was burning with enthusiasm to see an actual, living patient. At last the great day arrived. During his first lecture in internal medicine the instructor would show how a physician makes a diagnosis.

This initial presentation dealt with several patients in the earliest stages of a variety of infectious diseases. One at a time they were brought into the lecture room for the professor to question and examine. Selye noted with interest that the patients all seemed to fit into a rather general pattern. Each felt and looked ill, had a coated tongue, suffered various aches and pains, and complained of "stomach trouble" with accompanying loss of weight. Strangely, the professor dismissed these obvious signs of illness as though they were of little consequence.

At last the instructor called attention to what he really deemed important: the "characteristic" physical signs that would indicate precisely the specific disease developing in each patient. Selye, his eyes straining, leaned forward expectantly, but he concluded he must be too inexperienced to pick out these telltale signs. He was somewhat relieved when the teacher explained that in these particular patients most of the characteristic signs happened to be absent. Until they appeared there wasn't much a doctor could do, for without them it wasn't possible to determine accurately what disease the patient had.

Selye says, "It was clear that the many features of disease which were already manifest did not interest our teacher very much because they were 'nonspecific.' " [1] However, as a novice in the field of medicine the young student had a mind open to any possibilities. He understood the physician's need to pin down the specific disease so that precise treatment could be prescribed. But he was fascinated to note that many diseases initially make known their presence in the human body by producing symptoms common to other diseases. At that stage even an eminent professor couldn't tell one from the other.

Just plain sick

A clinical syndrome is "a group of symptoms and signs that occur together and characterize a disease." For instance, if a person experiences chills, headache, loss of appetite, fever, pain on chewing or swallowing, and swelling of the area below the ear, it is likely the doctor is going to say "mumps." It seemed significant to Selye that the patients brought before his class had a *collective* syndrome. Each might be on his way to developing a different disease, but at this stage all suffered a "just plain sick" syndrome. If it was important to find remedies for a particular disease, might it not be even more important to learn to deal with this "general syndrome of sickness."

Afraid of being laughed at, Selye never quite got up the courage to present his proposition to his physiology professor. Before long he was completely immersed in the physician's busy life of dealing with specific diseases, but tucked away in the back of his mind was the germ of an idea that would yet capture the attention of the entire world of medical science.

White rats and black despair

Ten years later young Dr. Selye turned to a career of academe and research in Montreal, and before long was surrounded by long rows of caged white rats. Persistent rumors of that day indicated the long-sought-for Fountain of Youth might actually soon be discovered. In laboratories around the world scientists were probing the mysteries of hormones and how they react in the human body. Professor Collip had assigned Selye the task of injecting an extract of cow's ovaries into rats whose ovaries or pituitary glands had been removed, to see what the hormonal effect might be.

As he did with anything he undertook, Selye gave himself completely to this project. When another all-night session seemed in the offing, his Scandinavian assistant, Kai Nielsen, would sometimes plead, "My heart has beat 30,000 times today, my blood has run 17 million miles, I have breathed 23,000 times, spoken about 4,000 words, moved 750 major muscles, and operated 14 billion brain cells. I am tired and you are too. Let's go home." Sometimes this approach worked in getting Selye to quit for the night.

At first the experiments seemed promising. All the test rats showed reactions that could not be obtained from injecting previously known sexual hormones. The animals' thymus gland and lymph nodes shrank, their adrenal glands became much larger, and they developed ulcers.

Selye was elated. "At the age of 28, I seemed already to be on the track of a new hormone. . . . It seemed only a matter of time now to concentrate and isolate the new hormone in pure form." [2] However, success proved to be coyly elusive.

As the young researcher worked on, doubts began to creep in. He discovered that his rats showed the same effects when he injected extracts of the kidney, spleen, or any other organ. Moreover, as he continually purified his extracts the results actually became *less* pronounced. The more impure his injections, the more potent they were. This certainly didn't seem to make much sense.

Bitter disappointment

Selye remembers one particularly dark, rainy afternoon in the spring of 1936. He was sitting in his small laboratory, brooding about the ever-increasing volume of findings that made it more and more improbable that his experimental substance could be a new hormone. Suddenly a horrible thought occurred. Perhaps all of the symptoms produced in the rats by his injections were merely owing to the impurity of his extracts. If that were true, all his work meant nothing.

As he reasoned, Selye's eyes fell on a bottle sitting on a shelf just in front of his desk. It contained Formalin, a highly irritating substance not derived from any living tissue. If his fears were well grounded, then even this fluid should produce the same reaction in his rats as the hormones had. Immediately he proceeded with this experimentation, and forty-eight hours later he carefully examined the organs of his animals. The answer was all too clear. There were the shrunken thymus glands and lymph nodes, the enlarged adrenals, and the ulcers. And the results were more pronounced than ever before.

The dreams of discovering a new hormone were shattered. Selye was so depressed that for days he was unable to work. He sat brooding in his laboratory, wondering what to do next.

Eventually he was inspired with a new thought: maybe it was possible to look at the test results from an entirely different angle. All of his various injections, from glandular extracts to Formalin, had produced the same *reaction* on the body organism. Perhaps an understanding of this syndrome or body response to injury might prove to be even more important than the discovery of a new hormone.

Then from the recesses of his mind came memories of that classroom scene some ten years earlier. He saw those patients in Prague with their coated tongues, vague aches and pains, stomach difficulties, loss of appetite, and general distress—all common symptoms that mark the beginning of many diseases. Selye had stumbled across the existence of a generalized reaction of the human body to many kinds of stress. His entire life since that time has been devoted to studying the effects of stress, helping people understand how it operates in their own experience. Anyone truly interested in achieving high-level wellness will want to give close attention to his findings.

What is stress?

Stress is simply the body's reaction to the wear and tear of life. Every single activity you engage in, every emotion you feel—whether it's asking the boss for a raise, getting badly sunburned, or competing in a foot race—sets up stress. And the way your body reacts to such stress agents, or "stressors," has much to do with your immediate health and your potential for a long life.

We need to understand just how the body responds to stress. Some years ago I made a solo foray into the jungle on the island of Espiritu Santo in the South Pacific. It was an altogether pleasant experience until I heard something moving through the underbrush, cutting across my path at a 45-degree angle. The "stressor" proved to be a large wild boar, sporting a wicked-looking set of tusks. I was aware of this creature's notoriously explosive temper and of what his sharp tusks can do to a hapless victim. Clearly this was a serious confrontation.

Under this stress situation certain of my bodily functions went into emergency gear in order to enable me to deal with the impending crisis. My adrenal glands, having received an alarm signal from my brain, began pumping adrenalin into my system to sharpen mental and physical faculties for either fight or flight. Although my hand had automatically gone to the handle of my sheath knife, a hand-to-hoof contest would have been hopelessly one-sided. An attempt at retreat through thick underbrush didn't appear to be a good option, either. Making like a rabbit, I did what seemed natural at the moment: I froze. Fortunately the wind was in my favor, and the beast trotted on by without ever suspecting he had company.

As soon as the danger was definitely past, my body quickly returned to its normal state. However, if the stress had been greatly prolonged, eventually I would have suffered complete exhaustion. Under extreme conditions stress itself can result in death.

Of course, a stressor doesn't have to be anything as fearful as a wild boar. It could be simply a family argument. Or some-

2

thing as gentle as a lover's kiss.

Actually it is not stress itself that is important or dangerous, but the mental and physical response to that stress. Fred Kerner in his book *Stress and Your Heart* says:

"Although you are constantly under strains of various kinds which keep you continually in a state of tension, you do not necessarily show stress symptoms because your mind and your body are working together to make the necessary, often automatic, adjustments. You breathe more deeply to replenish oxygen when it is needed. You sleep when you are tired. You eat when you are hungry. It is only when the strains imposed are excessive, or unexpected, or prolonged that serious symptoms of stress actually appear. If you should swallow a dose of poison for which there is no antidote, the strain is excessive. If you are struck a blow in the face, and are completely unprepared for it, the strain is unexpected. If you overwork yourself continuously, the strain is prolonged." [3]

Life's bank account

One of the most important discoveries in recent years is that each person is born with a certain amount of vital force with which to play out his life role. This amount varies from person to person. Selye describes it thus:

"It is as though, at birth, each individual inherited a certain amount of adaptation energy, the magnitude of which is determined by his genetic background. . . . There is just so much of it, and he must budget accordingly." [4]

In other words, the vital force we receive at birth is like a bank account from which we can make withdrawals at will, *but which we can never increase by making deposits.* The only control we have over this precious treasure is the rate at which we make our withdrawals.

Since stress is the wear and tear of life, people who tend to be spendthrifts of life's vital forces find themselves in difficulty.

"Health and physical fitness are treasures which one may possess in greater or lesser degree. No one is certain just how much of this treasure is at his disposal. Only when his withdrawals approximate an overdraft does he receive notice. This notice comes in the form of infections, degenerative diseases, fatigue, breathlessness, or weakness." [5]

Keeping the body under continual stress is like running an engine at high speed without letup. Eventually something has to give. When the body is stressed all parts are exposed to the tension, but whether it is the heart, the kidney, the stomach, or some other organ that breaks down depends on which organ happens to be the most vulnerable in that particular individual.

Speaking more generally, it is now believed that stress lays the foundation for some diseases, and aggravates many others.

Recently two California heart specialists linked our number one killer, heart disease, with the individual's response to stress. For twenty years Drs. Meyer Friedman and Ray Rosenman—director and associate director, respectively, of Mount Zion's Harold Brunn Institute—studied the relationship between personality and heart attacks. They suggest that individual personality traits play a much greater role in causing heart attacks than formerly suspected.

A high percentage of all patients having heart attacks under age 60 exhibit what these researchers term a "Type A" behavior pattern. Such individuals tend to be highly competitive and are constantly fighting the clock. In other words, their response to life keeps them in an almost continual state of stress. [6]

Is there any way to cheat?

What about burning the candle at both ends for short periods only, and then getting a bit of rest between spasms? Can we beat the game of life that way? Hans Selye checked this out carefully:

"Many people believe that, after they have exposed themselves to very stressful activities, a rest can restore them to where they were before. This is false. Experiments on animals have clearly shown that each exposure leaves an indelible scar, in that it uses up reserves of adaptability which cannot be replaced." [7]

Suppose John Smith keeps putting off figuring his annual income tax until the very last minute. Then he sits up nearly all night two nights in a row to meet that April 15 deadline. After another hard day at the office he comes home utterly exhausted. Without even bothering to eat he drops into bed and is immediately in a deep sleep. Since he doesn't have to be at work until noon the following day, his wife lets him sleep until he awakes by himself. Sixteen straight hours! After a shower and a good breakfast he feels as good as new again.

Actually John Smith is not quite as good as new. Fatigue is the body's built-in safety mechanism, and it kept him from destroying himself completely. But we don't bounce back from such a heavy stress situation without paying a price. John has drawn from his body's long-range reserves—reserves that no longer will be available at some later date.

When we follow John's reasoning we are like a spendthrift who happily keeps putting into his wallet dollars withdrawn from his bank account, without realizing that one day there won't be anything left to withdraw. Selye points out, "Since we constantly go through periods of stress and rest during life, just a little deficit of adaptation energy every day adds up—it adds up to what we call *aging.*"

Shall we vegetate?

Since any kind of activity produces at least some amount of wear and tear, it is obvious that complete freedom from stress does not exist. So it would seem the ideal program is conscientiously to avoid every possible bit of stress. Not so.

The most effective stress avoider I have ever met lives right under my own roof. Her name is Cookie, and she weighs in at about two pounds—soaking wet. The kind of "dog's life" she leads goes somewhat like this: I forcibly rout her out of her wicker bed just before I leave the house in the morning. While she is taking care of her duties in the back yard I fill her dishes with fresh food and water. Immediately upon being let back in the house, she hops into bed and is shut up in one room until we return in the evening. Upon our arrival home she cuts a few circles of uninhibited joy, but an hour later you would find her back in bed again. During an ordinary day—and most of her days are ordinary—she sleeps about 22 hours. Some who have to work unusually hard might be tempted to envy her "dog's life."

But although Cookie has been around several years, the tragedy is that she really has never lived at all. She merely exists. She has never been in a good dogfight, never had puppies, never gone to visit her relatives. The edge of her world is the perimeter of our yard. She did win a ribbon in an amateur dog show once, but I doubt she was aware of what was going on.

Attempting to avoid completely all forms of stress is not the answer. Research indicates too little activity also tends to shorten one's life-span.

While it is foolish to squander life by "burning out" at an early age, it is just as foolish to simply "rust out" while relatively young. As with most things in life, the secret is moderation and balance. Some of the happy things we do in life, such as taking a well-earned vacation, help prepare us for some of the greater stresses lying ahead.

Selye put it this way:

"Avoid stress whenever possible? Certainly not. Stress is the spice of life. . . . Who would enjoy a life of 'no runs, no hits, no errors'? Besides, certain types of activities have a curative effect and, actually, help to keep the stress mechanism in good shape." [8]

Let us spend wisely the precious treasure of vital force with which we have been endowed.

---

[1] Hans Selye, *The Stress of Life* (New York City: McGraw-Hill Book Company, Inc., 1956), p. 15.

[2] *Ibid.*, p. 22.

[3] Fred Kerner, *Stress and Your Heart* (New York City: Hawthorne Books Inc., 1961), p. 62.

[4] Selye, *op. cit.*, p. 66.

[5] Arthur H. Steinhaus, *Toward an Understanding of Health and Physical Education* (Dubuque, Iowa: Wm. C. Brown Co., 1963), p. 18.

[6] Meyer Friedman and Ray H. Rosenman, *Type A Behavior and Your Heart* (New York: Alfred A. Knopf, Inc., 1974).

[7] Selye, *op. cit.*, p. 274.

[8] Hans Selye, from an address to the National Conference on Fitness and Health (Canada, 1972).

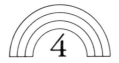

HOW
OLD ARE YOU—
FOR YOUR AGE,
THAT IS?

HAVE YOU ever had the privilege of entertaining a king and queen in your own home? I have, just once. Our royal guests were the Mir and Rani of the Shangri-La kingdom of Hunza. This pocket-sized principality (recently annexed by Pakistan) is tucked away in the high Himalayas where the borders of China, Afghanistan, and Pakistan converge. Although it can't be considered one of the great powers, Hunza is much in the news because of the longevity and freedom from disease enjoyed by its approximately 30,000 inhabitants.

Although reports sometimes have been exaggerated, it is true that the Hunzukuts are among the world's healthiest peoples. They not only live to unusual ages but remain vigorously active long after most of us are shuffling around at a snail's pace. The obvious question is "How come?"

Is one of their mountain springs the long-sought-for Fountain of Youth? Have they discovered some magic potion that could be exported to the rest of the world?

Life-style is the secret

There really is no great mystery. The answer can be summed up in one word—life-style. If we lived *where* the Hunzukuts live, and lived the *way* the Hunzukuts live, we would be able to match their state of well-being.

Locked in by the world's highest mountains, Hunza has been largely cut off from the rest of mankind for some 2,000 years. The rare visitors permitted to enter must endure a hair-raising air-cargo flight past intimidating peaks, followed by a tortuous jeep trip over "the world's most dangerous road." Only five feet wide in some places, this sole link with civilization could never be confused with an Interstate highway. Hung precariously on the steep mountain walls, it frequently presents a drop of some 3,000 or more nonstop feet down to the Hunza River. The sixty-eight-mile trip can be negotiated in a mere ten hours—provided one doesn't have to rebuild missing portions of the roadbed too often. It is no wonder Hunza has been deprived of most of the "benefits" modern civilization has to offer.

Frankly, the people of Hunza don't get much credit for their healthy condition. They live as they do largely because they have no choice. Their rather austere surroundings, for instance, dictate that they shall be temperate people. They like to refer to their country as "the land of just enough." By the same token, America could well be called "the land of just plain too much." Many of America's health problems are simply the result of overindulgence in the horn of plenty.

Take, for instance, the matter of exercise—or lack of it—an area where most of us would have to plead guilty. We buckle up our seat belts to drive two blocks for a loaf of bread. Not so the Hunzukut. For one thing, there aren't any cars to ride in; transportation is limited to foot power. Second, there are only two basic directions in the land of "Shangri-la"—up and down. To leave home and go anywhere is to indulge in a healthful form of exercise.

And when such exercise demands deep breathing, the Hunzukut doesn't suck in a draft of smog. Instead, his lung tissues are treated to an invigorating potion of clear, pristine, mountain air.

The water in Hunza is not laced with phosphates and industrial waste. It comes right off the melting glaciers, fresh and pure. There is some speculation that its mineral content may be highly beneficial.

The Hunzukuts are virtual vegetarians, as their limited tillable land has to be utilized for the production of food crops. On their terraced fields they raise grain, along with a wide variety of fruits, particularly apricots.

Perhaps most important of all, Hunza doesn't provide its inhabitants with a stressful environment. There are no hospitals, no drugstores, no army, no police force, no jails, no divorce, no traffic jams, and few if any clocks. People retire when the sun goes down, and they rise when it reappears. No newspapers or television stations inform the citizens what they should be worrying about during the next twenty-four hours. Wherever one goes in Hunza, one finds peace and quiet; there aren't even any dogs to bark at night. It truly is the land of just enough, and apparently of the right ingredients.

Thought provoking, isn't it? Sitting here in the midst of opulence, we might well wonder who should be feeling sorry for whom.

But what I'd like to point out just now is that each of us has two ages to take into account. First of all, there is our chronological age. We can't do very much about that. We were born on a certain day, and the pages of the calendar have been flipping by ever since. Those who are forever "thirty-nine and holding" are fooling no one but themselves.

There is also, however, the matter of our physiological age, and this we can do something about.

A few years ago the mail brought an invitation to attend the twentieth reunion of my high school graduating class. Although I was not able to attend, I did obtain a copy of the group photograph taken during the festivities. It was highly revealing. At the time of graduation we were all pretty much standardized: a group of teen-agers ready to set the world straight. But twenty years later we obviously had traveled various routes as far as physical well-being was concerned. Some "hadn't changed at all," while others appeared to be ready for early retirement.

What made the difference? Heredity has a part to play, of course, but perhaps the big factor was life-style. Let me demonstrate what I mean by sharing with you the actual experience of a personal friend.

Dr. Baker sheds twenty years

This friend, let's call him Dr. Baker, was more health conscious than the average person. When he dropped by the local YMCA for a stress test of heart function he did so with a fair degree of assurance. True, he was carrying around a few extra pounds, but he considered himself, generally speaking, a healthy specimen. The results of the test shook him up considerably. His resting pulse rate was 90 beats per minute; during a minute of exercise it shot up to 120 beats. The program director told it like it was: "Doctor, according to the test performance you are responding like a man ten years older than you really are. Results from the other tests we have run indicate premature aging. You'd better join our supervised exercise program."

This unsettling message reminded Dr. Baker that his own father had had his first heart attack at age 56 and died of another attack at 57. Two of his grandparents had passed away before the age of 60. It began to appear that if he intended to stay around much longer himself, it was time for decided action. He signed up for the YMCA conditioning program.

Week by week my friend faithfully followed the prescribed routine. Since he had no actual heart impairment, he was able to move along at a good pace. At the end of three months he was ready to repeat the original tests. Any inconvenience or unusual effort caused by the program was quickly forgotten when the results were in. Dr. Baker's resting pulse rate was now a steady 65, and his pulse after a minute of exercise was only 90, instead of 120. His heart action was now similar to the average man of 40 years. *Physiologically he had shed 20 years in only three months!* Dramatic? Definitely—and true.

I would like to point out again that a diseased heart would not have responded as quickly as did Dr. Baker's. He was not ill, but he was unfit. And continuing in an unfit condition eventually brings on illness of one kind or another. And so my friend turned his life around at the 50-year mark. Whatever your chronological age, you can do something significant about your physiological age if you really want to. Of course, the sooner you begin, the better.

Once you have a reasonable program under way, it is important to stay faithfully involved. Trained athletes have learned that two weeks of enforced rest may decrease their strength and ability to perform well by as much as 25 per cent. Unfortunately, however, getting back into a proper regimen doesn't close the gap in two weeks; it takes about six weeks to regain the lost ground. So conditioning must not be a casual, on-again-off-again affair, but rather a new way of life.

(Note: I just took a couple of minutes away from my writing to check my own resting pulse, and found it an encouraging 65 beats per minute. Why not lay this book down right now and check your own. If you don't like what you find, if your pulse is over 80, then it's time to take action. Nothing rash, however; obtain guidance from someone who can start you on a carefully controlled program.)

Climbing mountains at 78

So live a little! Don't sit feebly on the side lines while others are thoroughly enjoying the game of life. I know a fascinating young woman of 78, Hulda Crooks, who every year climbs to the top of Mount Whitney, at 14,495 feet the highest peak in the contiguous United States! A born athlete? Not at all. Early in life her health was so broken she was unable even to hold down a full-time job. Perennially tired and nervous, her circulation was so poor that for forty-five years she had to take two hot-water bottles to bed each night in order to keep warm. One was for her stomach and the other was for her feet. Always at midnight she had to get out of bed for a hot-water refill. At the age of 70 she began a careful but persistent program of outdoor running, and now the hot-water bottles are packed away for good. Or maybe she left them on Mount Whitney.[1]

China doctor

As I dialed the number from my motel room in Atlantic City, I thought about the fantastic gentleman I was planning to have interviewed on television. Dr. Harry Willis Miller, then in his ninety-first year, is the famed "China Doctor." Turning his back on a promising instructorship and practice in an American medical school, he has devoted almost his entire life to the Orient. He served as personal physician to nearly every one of China's heads of state, and while spending a few years in America raising funds for his projects, he was also consultant to two American Presidents, Taft and Wilson.

One of Dr. Miller's greatest contributions to mankind has been the development of soy milk. Countless babies owe their very life to this product that provides proper nutrition to youngsters unable to tolerate cow's milk. He also pioneered the soy-bean meat analogs, so much in the news today.[2]

A youthful voice answered the telephone, so I asked for the renowned physician. "This *is* Dr. Miller," came the firm, steady reply. I was dumbfounded. The voice just couldn't belong to a man in his nineties. But it did.

Dr. Miller's secret? A spare diet of the right foods, a love for walking rather than riding, and a real purpose in life. Here is a man so busy helping others that he just hasn't had time to grow old. Recognized as the prime mover in the raising up of numerous hospitals around the world, Miller started the most recent such project in Hong Kong at the age of 81. Ninety-six at the time of this writing, he is still busy converting dreams into reality.

How old are *you?* I hope people normally guess you younger than your chronological age, and not the other way around. If it's the latter, why not make a decision to change that picture, beginning today? You *can* do it, you know.

[1] Hulda Crooks, "Climbing Mountains at 76," in *Life and Health*, May, 1973, pp. 10-16.
[2] Raymond S. Moore, *China Doctor* (Mountain View, California: Pacific Press Publishing Assn., 1969).

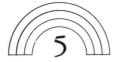

THREE
POUNDS OF
MIRACLES

I AM HOLDING a man-made miracle in the palm of my left hand. It is a rather innocent-looking little black box only three inches wide, five inches long, and one and one-half inches thick. In neat rows on its face are displayed some twenty buttons, and at one end a small window. Although packed with intricate circuitry, the miniature marvel weighs a mere nine and one-half ounces.

As I begin to play with the buttons, the innocent-looking little gadget comes alive. I punch the "7" button, and instantly that cipher appears glowing in the small window. A touch of the multiplication button, and immediately I'm told that 7 x 7 is 49. Another touch, and I learn that 7 x 49 is 343. Times 7 is 2,401. Times 7 is 16,807. Times 7 is 117,649. And so on, as fast as I can hit the button. Without a sound this little mathematical genius flashes back the answers, taking only 8/10ths of a second for each of its calculations. Fantastic. Other models, not much larger, can do complicated algebraic functions at a touch.

We stand in awe of today's electronic wizardry, and yet cradled securely within our own cranial cavity is a living computer so complex that its workings are beyond comprehension. The human brain is the most complicated mechanism we know.

It's electrical

As with most computers, the brain operates on electricity. You don't have to plug it into the wall, however, for the current is self-generated. My little hand-held calculator operates on dry cells, but your mind works more like a wet storage battery. One tenth of a volt of direct current is produced by a chemical reaction taking place within the brain cells. These electrical impulses are called brain waves, and your pattern is as unique to you as your fingerprint. Physicians often measure these brain waves to help diagnose certain neurological illnesses.

Consider your mind as the capital of your body. Your nervous system is like a complex telegraph network, constantly relaying messages at high speed. The individual nerve cells need only 1/1,000 of a second to rest before handling another signal, so these messages or nerve impulses can zip along through the body at speeds of nearly 200 miles per hour! And that's important when you have just touched your thumb to a hot griddle. The heat sensors in your thumb get the message, and reflex action causes you to remove your hand from the danger zone. Fortunately, this all happens very fast.

Because the nerve cells of the brain can communicate with other nerve cells through the proper routing of impulses, the agility of the human body is wonderful indeed. One physician, in a radio address, described the lightning calculations the brain must make to return a single ball during a tennis game: "The brain is able to survey and calculate data instant by instant as the ball changes speed, direction, and trajectory. The brain, with lightninglike speed, must calculate the probable point of impact, the intensity of the bounce, its future position in space, and the distance one must cover to make connection. It then goes through a similar complicated set of calculations to know at what angle to connect with the ball, how much force to put behind the racket in order to take advantage of the elasticity of the ball, and its subsequent flight through the air to hit the court in the most difficult spot for the opponent to return."

You can appreciate the immense complexity of all this only if you remember the virtual storm of signals that continually assault the human mind. Messages having to do with heat, cold, pain, pressure, equilibrium, light, sound, smell, et cetera. Such a barrage might be expected to blow a fuse, but normally the mind sorts everything out, takes appropriate action, and even stores information away for future use—no more bare fingers on hot griddles.

We still understand little about what goes on within the mind's more than 12 *billion* cells. We suppose that we feel with our fingers, see with our eyes, and hear with our ears, but actually all this takes place within the brain itself. Our fingers, eyes, and ears merely gather raw data to be interpreted elsewhere.

An infinite filing system

Perhaps most awe inspiring of all is the fact that the mind seems to have an infinite capacity for storing information. It seems that everything you experience from birth onward is filed away in the inner recesses of your mind, as though on magnetic tape. Some of it is not available for instant replay—you have "forgotten" about it. But the information is there, nevertheless, and under certain types of stimulation it can be recalled. Millions upon millions of detailed memories are faithfully filed away in a tiny storage cabinet, weighing only three pounds and taking up less space than a shoe box!

An intimate relationship

The arriving guests found a table that had been carefully set. The food itself was nourishing and well prepared. Although the dinner conversation was warm and spirited, by the time the meal was over all participants were thoroughly sick. Several even vomited the meal they had barely finished.

The difficulty? Nothing more than a few drops of food coloring. The meat served was a bilious green, the milk a bright blue, and the butter a chocolate brown. Other equally weird color combinations graced the table; nothing looked familiar. Past experience told the diners when the meat is green it is best left strictly alone, and who could guess the horrors hidden in a serving of bright-red mashed potatoes. Although the participants knew the food was perfectly safe, no one was able to put mind over matter.

The important lesson to be learned from this interesting experiment is that the mind and the body are intimately related. When one is affected, the other sympathizes. In other words, the state of the mind has to do with the health of the body—and a diseased or much-abused body also has a telling effect on the mind.

As far back as Hippocrates, the Father of Medicine, it was recognized that man's emotions could produce certain physical effects. But it was not until A.D. 1818 that Heinroth coined the word that is often used to describe this phenomenon, "psychosomatic" disease. The Greek word for mind is *psuche* and that for the body is *sōma*. So we are dealing now with "mind-body" disease.

How prevalent is this manifestation? Dr. Samuel Silverman, associate professor of psychiatry at Harvard Medical School, believes that with *all* illnesses there is an interaction between the emotions and the body. It is almost certain that everyone, whether he knows it or not, has had an emotionally induced illness at one time or another. Let me speak as one who does know.

A pain in the back

While working in Pakistan I came under severe emotional stress that continued without interruption for some time. Although the situation was unavoidable, I thought I was handling it reasonably well. However, it was during this period I began to experience a sharp pain in my back. Highly localized, the affected spot was about one inch from my spinal column and perhaps the size of a dime. Because the pain persisted, I decided to see a doctor about it.

The physician seemed to have difficulty diagnosing my problem. Heat treatments didn't help, and neither did massage. The next procedure was to be an injection directly into the trouble area, but before my benefactor could schedule this procedure I left for a vacation in the fabled Vale of Kashmir. This lush valley, crisscrossed with canals and completely ringed by towering snow-covered peaks, is right out of the storybooks. A person would have to work hard to retain his problems amid such peaceful surroundings.

My tent had been pitched for only a day or two when I suddenly realized I no longer had a pain in my back. Having read about psychosomatic illness, I realized what had taken place. I was fascinated that such a genuine pain could originate completely in the mind. Now that I was an "expert" on the subject, I was sure I could never be so easily tricked again. How wrong I was.

A few months later, with the same stress problem still complicating my days, I developed a pain in my left leg. Nothing excruciating; just a steady dull, nagging ache. Before I was able to get it diagnosed and treated, an assignment took me to a very remote area some twenty miles beyond the farthest police outpost. I began my journey on a large air liner, changed to a smaller plane, then to a large river steamer, next to a small launch, and finally to a jungle footpath. We never know how busy and frantic our workaday world really is until we contrast it with real peace and quiet. Forty-eight hours after arriving at my destination I no longer had an ache in my left leg. Again my body had been sympathizing with my mind.

So, you see, when one labels someone else "a pain in the neck," he may be more accurate than he realizes. The great physician Sir William Osler once said, "It is much more important to know what sort of patient has a disease than what sort of disease a patient has."

You may be wondering, "But why a pain in the left leg? Why not the right? If I suffer similar stress how do I know it won't show up as a throbbing in my big toe, or even a case of blurred vision?" You can't know. However, certain clues sometimes predict those places where psychosomatic illness could strike.

Proneness to specific diseases?

As mentioned in chapter 3, twenty years of study have convinced Drs. Friedman and Rosenman that more than 90 per cent of all heart attack victims exhibit a behavior pattern they label "Type A." Such persons have a compelling sense of urgency— "hurry sickness." They tend to be aggressive and competitive, with a marked amount of free-floating hostility. Type A's engage in a chronic struggle against circumstances, against others, against themselves. The researchers estimate that half of all American males—and a growing percentage of females—are more or less confirmed Type A's.[1]

Dr. Silverman states that "when a person develops 'critical stress' and cannot cope, . . . either the mind or body breaks down. If physical illness strikes, 'it doesn't do so randomly, but at vulnerable spots unique for each of us.' Where the physical illness shows up 'depend[s] on which organs have been "sensitized" by heredity, childhood diseases, or [one's own] neurotic strategies.' "[2]

It is thought that emotional stress affects the body systems in two general ways. Emotions linked with hostility cause these systems to overreact, while attitudes such as fear or sadness result in underreaction. Often these reactions are temporary and mild in nature. Fear of making a public speech may cause the palms of our hands to sweat; if we become embarrassed, blood may rush to our face and we blush. Such reactions are not particularly significant, but if the stress is prolonged, then consequences can be serious. Some of the illnesses that may be caused by emotional stress are duodenal ulcer, chronic indigestion, ulcerative colitis, hypertension (chronic high blood pressure), and attacks of bronchial asthma.

How to avoid trouble

Are we helpless, then, against the onslaughts of emotionally induced disease—mere pawns in the game of life? Not at all; there is much we can do to avoid this type of difficulty. Because the mind is the capital of the body, proper decision-making here can be beneficial throughout the body.

3

Evidence indicates viruses do not begin their destructive work on the human body until a physical or chemical irritant gives them their chance. In other words, people who are *generally* unfit are less able to withstand stress without complications. If you want to avoid trouble, try to keep yourself in top physical condition at all times. This is "frustrating" to germs.

It is also wise to avoid situations apt to place you under emotional tension. Counting to ten may not be such a bad idea, after all. A few hours after avoiding an angry confrontation the original problem may seem trivial and hardly worthy of attention. If it seems you simply must "get it off your chest" (another interesting psychosomatic phrase) try writing it all out in great detail in a letter. Then instead of mailing the letter, toss it into the wastebasket.

Learn to recognize unsuspected sources of emotional stress. Dr. Allan Magie says, "When subjected to unexpected bursts of either momentary or steady-state *noise*, the human body responds with the same kind of reactions experienced during emotional states such as anger or fear. The specialist terms them stress or arousal responses. Changes occur in breathing, pulse rate, secretion of hormones, blood pressure, digestive functions, and other body responses." [3]

We seldom realize the noise level created by our modern technology. There is the continual hum, clank, or roar of the dishwasher, street traffic, food blender, vacuum cleaner, passing jetliner, lawn mower, and blare of radio and TV. We may consider this merely "background" noise, but scientists are realizing more and more the serious consequences it can have on the human system. It is wise to avoid as much din as possible.

We also can be alert to situations particularly fraught with danger. It has been observed that serious illness is often preceded by a significant life crisis. The emotional shock most difficult to adjust to seems to be that caused by the death of a spouse. Not only can such a traumatic experience bring on sickness but the duration of that illness is often determined by the attitude of the bereaved person.

By the way, don't ever be deluded into thinking you may

be helped with some problem by allowing yourself to be hypnotized. Don't turn the "capital" of your body over to any other human power. Under a hypnotic trance the subconscious mind of one person is controlled by another, and the result is often an *increased* state of emotional imbalance and dependency. This is an area fraught with real danger.[4]

Unrecognized power

We have yet to realize the power of the mind. Until only recently we assumed certain bodily functions were controlled by the involuntary nervous system, and therefore were totally beyond our conscious control. Now we know that this is not entirely true. Some individuals have demonstrated a remarkable ability to change their heart rate, systolic blood pressure, and temperature of their hands, merely through concentration. It follows, then, that by proper exercise of the will we can help keep our bodies functioning as they should. We are not mere playthings at the mercy of fate. We are God-formed men and women with the ability to make intelligent choices. We have the privilege of shaping our own attitudes.

Many physicians can testify to the authority of the will. Two patients may be suffering from the same disease. One simply gives up and, in spite of all that modern medicine has to offer, passes away. The other individual refuses to surrender. He summons all his mental energies to his aid, and with the help of his physician fights his way back to a state of good health. If it is true that diseases have emotional components, is it not simple logic that the mind should also be instrumental in helping throw off disease?

Think positive

Probably nothing promotes ill health as much as an undue concern with one's self. We can turn our thoughts inward to the extent we become mental cripples—with physical crippling sure to follow. Some lifelong invalids could have been happy and well if they had only thought so. The best way to forget your own problems is by losing yourself in service for others.

You'll be surprised how your own difficulties will melt away.

Remember, then, to think positively. Solomon, perhaps the wisest man who ever lived, said, "A cheerful heart does good like medicine, but a broken spirit makes one sick" (Prov. 17:22, T.L.B.).[5] One survey indicated that those who live longest are those who enjoy their work the most. Will Rogers had it pretty well figured out when he said, "Most people are about as happy as they make up their mind to be."

Just as negative thoughts may destroy us, so positive attitudes will help us maintain optimum health. The following are two lists that may prove helpful in reminding you what to avoid and what to strive for:

Can Produce Illness	Will Promote Good Health
Depression	A sense of satisfaction
Guilt	A consciousness of rightdoing
Distrust	Cheerfulness
Selfishness	Courage
Sadness	Hope
Anxiety	Faith
Discontent	Sympathy
Grief	Love
Remorse	Usefulness
Anger	Gratitude
Fear	Trust
Envy	Calmness
Frustration	Contentment
Jealousy	Service for others

Why not set your mind right now? Determine to rise above life's difficulties and to have a long, healthy, happy life.

[1] Meyer Friedman, M.D., and Ray H. Rosenman, M.D., *Type A Behavior and Your Heart* (New York: Alfred A. Knopf, 1974), pp. 67-70.

[2] Samuel Silverman, *Time*, Sept. 30, 1974, p. 65.

[3] Allan Magie, Ph.D., "Quiet Please," *Life and Health*, March, 1973, pp. 14-17.

[4] H. Jacobsen, *Modern Treatment of Tense Patients* (Springfield, Illinois: Charles C. Thomas Publishers, 1970), p. XIV (introduction).

[5] All Bible texts credited to T.L.B. are from *The Living Bible, Paraphrased* (Wheaton: Tyndale House Publishers, 1971). Used by permission.

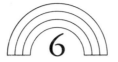

ALLOWING
YOUR BODY TO
DO ITS OWN
THING

"IF YOU'RE going to fix the windshield wipers on the Pontiac, why don't you have Craig help you? It's good for teenagers to learn something about taking care of a car."

My wife was speaking, and at the time her suggestion seemed not only logical but commendable. Cornering my son before he could escape through the back door, I steered him toward the driveway. Within minutes I was experiencing that sense of satisfaction that comes to a man when he has a wrench in his hand and grease on his face.

You probably know that if your windshield wipers have been caught in midcycle, turning on your automobile's ignition key will cause them to return immediately to home base. If you are the parent of a teen-ager you also know that this particular species can't go for more than a few minutes without musical input—the louder the better. I was completely preoccupied with my work when my son slid behind the wheel and turned the ignition key so as to be able to operate the radio. Faithfully the wiper mechanism completed its cycle. Unfortunately, my little finger was positioned right on home base.

Had the appendage been turned ever so slightly, it would have been completely guillotined at the first joint. Instead the

knifelike edge of the wiper mechanism made a neat surgical
incision approximately one inch in length. In the second or
two before blood filled the wound I was treated to a brief lesson in anatomy. Clearly visible were bone, muscle, tendons,
fat, and a couple of other items unrecognizable to a layman.
Dripping blood, I left for the emergency room with my son
driving. For once he didn't turn the radio on.

The emergency room was top notch. In no time at all my
injured finger was anesthetized, carefully washed, soaked in
disinfectant, and sewn up with tiny sutures. A tetanus shot
came as a bonus. But impressive as the medical care was, the
real miracle began as I left the emergency-room door.

Skyscrapers are easy

We take so much for granted in this world, such as the
"simple" healing of a wound. The truth is that even the tiniest
cut calls for a reconstruction job far more complex than the
building of a New York skyscraper. Except for this amazing
body process there would be no practice of surgery, and even
the slightest injury could result in death.

If a wound is relatively severe the body immediately goes
on full alert to meet the crisis. Blood pressure drops to keep
the loss of blood at a minimum. Blood clotting, which in test
tubes takes three or four minutes, now takes place in a few
seconds. The spleen empties its reserve supply of blood into
the system to help replace what has been lost. The white-
blood-cell count goes up to fight infection.

Our body cells are constantly bathed in fluid, but a wound
exposes them to the drying effect of air. This is a problem that
has to be corrected immediately. Lymph, tissue juices, and
plasma flood into the wound site to provide the necessary
moisture. At the same time the flow of blood must somehow
be stanched.

Blood normally resists clotting because a blood clot in the
circulatory system can result in serious injury or death. But
when a wound opens up, the blood must instantly reverse its
usual characteristic and clot. Platelets, which are always pres-

ent in the blood stream, clump together in the presence of a substance called *thromboplastin,* which is released by injured tissue. This starts the formation of a clot. Further complex chemical reactions produce *fibrin.* This white, cottonlike material traps red blood cells, thus forming a lifesaving stopper. It also plugs up the ends of exposed lymphatic ducts so that dangerous bacteria cannot sneak into the body by this route.

Minute blood vessels near the edge of the wound have already begun to dilate. Their walls eventually become so porous the white blood cells can escape. These little scavengers literally eat up anything that might slow the healing process such as bacteria, dead cells, or dirt. They finally gobble up so many of the invading organisms that they themselves die. If there is pus in a wound, it is made up of these sacrificed white cells.

Reconstruction gets under way

Thus far we have spoken only about measures designed to meet the emergency. Next the important job of reconstruction gets under way. A major role in this process is played by the *fibroblasts,* specialized cells that develop in the wound site. By attaching themselves to the cottony fibrin, they fill the wound with a temporary patch. The blood vessels that normally bring nourishment to the cells are disrupted at the time of the injury. However, these fibroblasts have the ability to absorb their food directly from the fluid in the wound itself. Within a few days they will have established themselves so firmly they no longer need the framework provided by the fibrin. The latter is then dissolved to provide additional nourishment for cell growth.

Now the wound begins to fill with a spongy material called *granulation tissue* composed of fibroblasts, capillaries, and white blood cells. As the tiny little blood vessels begin to grow into the area, their ends are sealed so that precious blood cells will not leak away. Eventually the sealed ends dissolve and link up into a brand-new circulatory system. So that feeling too can be restored, a network of nerve endings also advances into the affected area.

Skin cells around the edge of the wound begin to multiply and reach toward the center. The first layer of new skin to cover the wound is thin, fragile, and living. As it matures the uppermost cells will die and form a harder, more permanent covering.

When the scab drops away revealing new skin beneath, one is apt to remark, "Look, it's all healed up. I'm as good as new." Actually, the entire healing process may take many more months. Injured muscle tissue must heal, and fatty tissue and connective tissue must be restored. Finally the reparative connective tissues are replaced by normal, functioning tissue. Perhaps a year has passed, and now the miracle of healing is truly complete.[1]

The "simple" healing of a wound? One of the greatest army surgeons of all time, Ambroise Paré (1510-1590), felt he played only a small role in an incomprehensible mystery. Inscribed in French on the base of a statue erected in his honor is this humble philosophy: "I treated him, God healed him."

My own minor wound was cut so neatly, cared for so quickly, and kept so free from infection that it healed by what is called "first intention." Now, three months later, my finger is so completely healed I can hardly tell where the skin was damaged. Occasionally I hear people discussing the possibility of "divine healing." Really, *is there any other kind?*

The cost of impatience

If nature has such wonderful restorative powers, why aren't most people in better health? In pondering this question, let's remember that disease is merely nature's effort to free the system from conditions resulting from a violation of the laws of health. The first step should be to find out *why* one is sick, and the second, to work intelligently to remove the cause. If sitting on a tack causes pain, it would seem a most logical and proper response would be to get up and remove the tack.

Sometimes we know perfectly well the source of our problem, but we are unwilling to take whatever steps are necessary to alleviate the condition. Certain poor health habits may need altering. And that would call for a change in life-style, a cranking up of the will power. It's much easier to plead with a physician for a bottle of pills or an injection to ease the symptoms. We postpone facing up to the actual cause until some future date.

Impatience is another factor. Nature's way of doing things seems entirely too slow. Many want immediate relief from the pain and inconvenience brought on by disease. Again the answer seems to lie in a needle or a bottle.

We have become a nation of pill takers. Annually we spend a staggering amount on the brightly colored little capsules and tablets that promise so much—more than 3 billion dollars on prescription pills alone. We gobble them to keep us awake, to put us to sleep, to make us lose weight, to make us gain weight, to slow us down, to speed us up; a pill for every purpose.

Some, particularly young people, have found there's a thrill in the pill. Popping a handful of them can result in a chemical high that blows one's mind—literally. These popular drugs have left a wide trail of permanent mind damage, broken health, accidental death, and suicide. Very expensive kicks.

Years ago popular nostrums included such poisonous ingredients as strychnine, arsenic, mercury, and opium. They could be purchased at any drug counter without a prescription, and were popularly used for even minor ailments. Although they sometimes seemed to provide a measure of relief, all too often their long-range harvest was convulsions, paralysis, and death.

Today's potent drugs

The Federal Drug Administration has taken these old-time killers off the market, but we still need to have a healthy respect for today's powerful medicines. Scores of new drugs are introduced each year and, although certain testing programs are compulsory, we do not know all the possible effects the drugs may have on the human system, for some do not become evident until some later date.

We still recoil at the horror of the thalidomide tragedy, when pregnant mothers who used the drug gave birth to pitifully misshapen offspring. In West Germany alone, 3,000 living children have only seallike flippers for arms and legs because their mothers used this potent medicine. Who is to say such a thing couldn't happen again? After all, it took us 80 years to learn that common aspirin can cause bleeding from the surface of the stomach wall. And literally tons of it are consumed each day.

In the strictest sense, drugs do not cure disease. At best they merely assist nature in her restorative work. Drugs are used to suppress uncomfortable symptoms until the natural processes effect a cure. A few drugs may actually hinder the healing process, or merely change the form or location of the illness. "One of the most commonly prescribed tranquilizers listed in the American Medical Association's edition of *New Drugs* has the following possible side effects: drowsiness, dizziness, fatigue, lack of muscular coordination, nausea, blurred vision, seeing double, low blood pressure, headaches, impairment of memory, slurred speech, tremor, rash, involuntary voiding, constipation, and paradoxic reactions such as excitement, depression, stimulations, and hallucinations. Other cautions are that the drug should be avoided or used with care by persons with psychotic tendencies, impaired liver or kidney function, glaucoma, or in conjunction with certain antidepressants (mood elevators)." [2]

Dr. Kenneth L. Melmon, professor of clinical pharmacology at the University of California, says that "3 to 5 per cent of patients admitted to the hospital are there because of drug reactions. . . . Eighteen per cent to 30 per cent of hospital patients will have a bad reaction to a drug given while they are hospitalized." [3]

Difficulty brought on by the drug itself occasionally can be much worse than the original problem. Carl R. Kjeldsberg states flatly, "There is really no nontoxic drug. . . . In the

United States in 1957, allergy to penicillin alone caused approximately 1,800 deaths." [4] Nature is often called to a double task: to fight the effects of the drugging along with the disease itself. Many times a perceptive physician will take a patient off all medications, allowing the body to regain its strength and mend itself in its own natural way.

I am not suggesting all medications are bad, but only that they should be used sparingly and with professional guidance. Let me relate a personal experience to illustrate my point.

A personal experience

Some months ago I found myself suffering high fever and violent chills. These periodic attacks seemed to lack other symptoms that might be associated with the prevalent "flu bug." The doctor I visited listened to my history and checked me over, but was unable to come up with any specific diagnosis. He prescribed a strong, broad-spectrum antibiotic, hoping this would take care of whatever was ailing me. This could be called a "shotgun approach."

The attacks of fever and chills continued, and eventually I consulted another physician. His approach was interesting. After examining me carefully, he said, "I don't know what's wrong with you, so I'm not going to do anything at all right now. But when you spike a fever again, come to the hospital right away. We'll run some tests to find out the cause of your problem. Then we'll be able to do something to change the picture."

The doctor found that playing Sherlock Holmes for my case wasn't easy. I was in the hospital for ten days and underwent numerous tests. One by one, the possibilities were eliminated until the actual trouble was pinpointed. I had contracted typhoid in Southern Asia eleven years previously, was treated, and considered cured. Actually, some of the typhoid germs had hidden away in my gall bladder and remained dormant there for more than a decade. Now, for some unknown reason, they had begun showering out into my blood stream, causing the fever and chills. I was thankful to learn what was wrong before the situation grew even more serious.

By the way, if I had learned about my problem a few years earlier, I would now be walking around minus my gall bladder, for that was the prescribed treatment then. But recently certain antibiotics have been developed that are specific for this problem, and my physician felt the use of such medications was indicated. This was a "rifle" rather than a "shotgun" approach. The treatment proved to be effective, according to later tests, and I have never had any difficulty along that line since. I for one am thankful that the research laboratories came up with a medication that not only relieved my symptoms but also helped effect a permanent cure.

The better way

Allow the laws of nature to operate in your favor. The natural way to healing may seem slower, but in the long run it is best. Select a physician who will work with you in this effort. Don't push him to prescribe a quick remedy; instead, let him know you want to use medications only when he feels they are positively indicated.

And best of all, learn for yourself more about nature's marvelous healing powers. Seek to find the cause of your difficulty, and then strike at the root of the problem. Cooperate with nature in her effort to re-establish balance and harmony in your body systems. Finally, learn all you can about nature's own true remedies. They are so important we are going to devote an entire chapter to each one of them: pure air, sunlight, abstemiousness, rest, exercise, water, and a proper diet.

---

[1] J. D. Ratcliff, "The Wonder of a Healing Wound," *Reader's Digest*, September, 1959, pp. 169-172.

[2] Harry Spizman, "A Caution for Prescription Drugs," *Life and Health*, March, 1975, p. 18.

[3] *Ibid.*, p. 19.

[4] Carl R. Kjeldsberg, "Iatrogenic Disease," *Pathobiology*, Minckler, Anstall, and Minckler (St. Louis, Mo.: C. V. Mosby Co., 1971), pp. 172, 173.

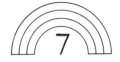

A BREATH OF
FRESH AIR

WE HAD spent a delightful week on a ranch in the high reaches of the San Jacinto Mountains east of Los Angeles. The sky had been blue, the sun brilliant, the air cool and bracing. No one really wanted to leave, but according to the calendar it was time to face up to workaday life once again.

As we cleared the highest point in the road and began to dip toward the valley, we could hardly believe the sickening vista before us. Half-way down the mountain a sea of thick, dirty, yellow smog stretched west as far as one could see toward the Pacific Ocean. It didn't seem that air-breathing creatures should venture into such a noxious mixture, but civilization lay somewhere beneath it, and that is where salary checks come from. The smog level was so well defined we almost expected to feel a slight "bump" as our automobile made its re-entry.

The pollution that plagues our cities today is a real tragedy, because fresh, invigorating air is one of nature's best remedies. Just as fish live in the depths of the ocean, so human beings live at the bottom of the sea of air that envelops the earth. We can go weeks without food, days without water, but only a few minutes without air.

Air consists of a combination of several different gases. Oxygen, the vital one for man, makes up one fifth of the total volume. We carry about two quarts of oxygen in our blood, lungs, and body tissues—enough to last approximately four minutes.

Every activity we engage in requires energy, and our bodies produce this energy by burning the "fuel" present in living cells. This fuel is derived from the food we eat; the flame that consumes it is oxygen. If our supply of this life-sustaining gas is cut off for more than a few minutes disaster follows immediately. Our brain, our heart, everything, ceases to function. We take altogether too lightly our need for pure air, with its precious cargo of oxygen.

Since everyone is busy breathing 24 hours a day, we might wonder when the world is going to run out of oxygen. Providentially, the earth's plant life absorbs the carbon dioxide we breathe out, and in turn gives off oxygen. It is estimated that algae in the ocean provide almost 90 per cent of the oxygen in our atmosphere, with the rest coming from plants on land.[1]

In humans, the exchange of oxygen and carbon dioxide takes place in our lungs. These spongelike organs contain about 600 million tiny air sacs, with walls so thin (only one cell thick) that oxygen molecules can pass right through them and unite with the hemoglobin in our red blood cells. When our blood absorbs this life-giving substance it turns a bright red.[2]

The brain most easily affected

The body cells most easily affected by a lack of oxygen are those of the brain, particularly the higher centers that deal with reason, will power, judgment, and emotion. We know that when a person is completely deprived of oxygen he dies. We also need to understand that a person partially starved for oxygen is "half dead." If mountain climbers ascend into the thin air of higher altitudes without oxygen tanks they begin to get clumsy, are easily confused, and are extremely grouchy and irritable.

Most of us never come even close to taking advantage of our natural lung capacity. We are shallow breathers, using only the top portion of our lungs. Why not stop right now and concentrate on expelling every bit of air from the farthest reaches of your lungs. Now then, take in all the air your lungs can possibly hold. Come on, just a little bit more. Now go through this cycle several times. You may feel a bit light-headed because your body may not be used to expelling carbon dioxide so quickly. Continue to practice deep breathing. Keep at it until proper breathing becomes second nature.

Beware of poor posture, for stooping or sitting in a slouch makes deep breathing almost impossible. Improper respiration results in drowsiness and susceptibility to disease. Shallow breathing not only has an adverse effect on the lungs; the stomach, liver, and brain are also affected. On the other hand, good respiration soothes the nerves, stimulates the appetite, and induces sound, refreshing sleep.

Mouth breathing should also be avoided, as the nose has been designed to control the temperature and humidity of air entering the lungs. Since nasal membranes are covered with mucus and hairlike filaments, the nose also filters out foreign particles that would otherwise end up in the lungs.

Ventilation is important

Proper ventilation of the home is also important to good health. Inasmuch as impurities from the lungs and the pores of the skin are continually being absorbed by the air around us, it obviously is not good to breathe the same air over and over again. (An exception might be during a smog alert, when it would be better to recycle the inside air. It would be well if you have an air conditioner with an activated charcoal filter.) If at all possible, rooms should be thoroughly aired each day. Particularly is this true of sleeping rooms. Years ago, night air was considered positively dangerous, but now we know better. Open your bedroom windows, summer and winter. You'll wake up more refreshed in the morning and better able to face the day's program.

Count your blessings if you live out in the country where air is still relatively pure. Last summer I saw cyclists in the city peddling along with masks over their faces. Before long we may step up to a coin-operated machine and buy a measure of oxygen as casually as we now purchase a package of peanuts.

It's about time we all take note of what is happening to the only "ocean" of air we have to live in. A few years ago my family vacationed in the beautiful Adirondack Mountains of upper New York State, and enjoyed the pristine forest air. Since then particulates in that mountain air have increased tenfold, because the area is upwind of the great cities of the East. There is evidence that some chronic bronchitis, emphysema, cancer, and allergies are in part a result of air-pollution problems.[3]

The greatest single culprit in polluting our planet's air supply is that chrome-plated, gas-guzzling behemoth of the highway, the much beloved American automobile. Microparticulates (especially small particles) are not filtered out by respiratory hairs or mucus, so they may become lodged in our lung tissue or pass right into our blood stream. An idling auto may emit as many as *one hundred billion microparticulates per second*. Some 2 million tons of polluting particles are suspended in the world's atmosphere already. If our present high rate of increase of air pollution continues unabated, by A.D. 2040 we will be able to boast 228 million tons as a permanent load. Such a large-scale shroud around the earth would have a dire effect on global weather patterns.[4]

We are each partly responsible for what is happening to our precious air. Whenever we can do something to help change this dismal picture, we should do so. In the meantime, let's practice filling our lungs to capacity with the freshest air available.

[1] *The Wonderful Human Machine* (Chicago, Illinois, 1971), American Medical Association, p. 25.

[2] *Ibid.*, p. 28.

[3] Rosalyn Kane and George A. Wistreich, *Biology for Survival* (Beverly Hills: Glencoe Press, 1974), pp. 255, 256.

[4] Henry A. Schroeder, *The Poisons Around Us* (Bloomington, Indiana: Indiana University Press, 1974), p. 4.

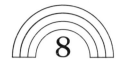

MAN IS SOLAR
POWERED

FROM ANCIENT times men have stood in awe of the giant furnace that dominates our solar system. The entire surface of the sun is in constant agitation, erupting and casting massive sheets of flame 20,000 to 30,000 miles into space, with an occasional jet of fire reaching out a million miles.[1] Scientists still do not comprehend the source of such unlimited heat. If the surface of the sun were completely covered with ice to a depth of fifty feet, this frigid shell would melt away in a mere sixty seconds! [2]

But the sun is more than heat and light. It is a never-failing reservoir of energy, ultimately necessary to life for every living thing on earth. Plants depend on sunlight for their growth, and man himself is solar powered. Our space probes capture light from the sun, converting it into electrical energy to operate small motors. In a similar manner plants capture the sun's energy; then we eat those plants to obtain energy fuel to operate our muscles.

Sunlight is a healing balm; it has the ability to kill germs. Sunshine on the skin helps produce vitamin D. And the sun's infrared rays are good for various aches and pains. The soothing heat increases circulation, removes waste, and helps tense muscles to relax.

4

Earlier we mentioned the healthy Hunzukuts who remain vigorous even though advanced in years. Interestingly enough, their near neighbors to the south are not nearly so robust. The explanation seems to be that even in wintertime Hunza still gets ample sunshine, while in neighboring Nagir the mountains are situated so as to cut off most of the sun's rays. Some portions of Nagir receive no more than twenty minutes of sunshine during the shortest days of the year.

Animals seem to know instinctively that the sun's rays are beneficial. Our Chihuahua dog, Cookie, spends the day moving from one position on the carpet to another, so as always to be in a patch of sunlight.

When building a home, it is good to avoid low, damp areas, and to seek high ground where each room in the house can have plenty of sunlight. Vines and shade trees are admittedly attractive, but they should not be positioned so as to cut off the sun's rays. Sunlight may eventually fade the carpets and the draperies, but it will put color in the cheeks of our children.

To broil or not to broil

It should be kept in mind that sunshine is strong medicine, and it's possible to have too much of a good thing. Years ago milady took stringent measures to keep her milky white complexion from being contaminated by Old Sol. Not so today. Modern maidens and their male escorts begin their lemminglike rush to the seashore with the first warm days of spring and summer. A deep tan may be all the rage as far as fashion is concerned, but if you don't like freckles, sunspots, dry, rough skin, or wrinkles, then don't overdo the sun-bathing. Temperance again. Remember that a reasonable amount of sunlight is necessary if we are to remain strong and free of disease.

---

[1] Phillip L. Knox, *Today's Amazing Universe* (Nashville, Tennessee: Southern Publishing Association, 1953), pp. 43-49.
[2] Walter J. Rich, *The Message of the Stars* (Nashville, Tennessee: Southern Publishing Association, 1950), pp. 18-23.

9

FEAST OR FAST?

THE OTHER day my son received a thirty-five-dollar lesson in the form of a motorcycle repair bill. On the ticket the shop foreman had written, "The engine had twice as much oil in it as the manual calls for." Apparently my son had concluded that if something is good for a machine, then twice as much has to be even better. It didn't turn out that way.

The human body is actually a chemical engine, operating on the energy we get from our food. If we insist on putting in the wrong kind of fuel (food), or in overloading the system, with too much, even of a good thing, we can expect some kind of "engine trouble."

One of nature's finest allies is abstemiousness. Ordinarily I would avoid a fourteen-letter word, but in this case it seemed to be the only one saying exactly what I wanted. It simply means "eating and drinking sparingly."

Special occasions are often used as an excuse for overeating. Many seem unable to push themselves away from the festive board until they have eaten themselves into a lethargic stupor. Their digestive system is completely bogged down with the overload. Others eat as though they consider *every* day a holiday. This kind of abuse is often the unsuspected cause of illness.

Resting the stomach

In many cases of sickness, the best possible remedy is simply to fast for a meal or two, letting the organs of digestion have a chance to rest. A high fever often can be brought down by abstaining from food for a short time. Of course, if food is withheld for too long a time the patient becomes enfeebled. When the fever breaks light nourishment should be given.

Fruit is easily digested; some have found relief from distress by switching to a fruit diet for a few days. Going without any food (taking only water) for a day or two has proved beneficial even for some who are not ill, particularly if employed in a sedentary occupation.

Of course, it is possible to overdo a good thing, and right now fasting seems to be a fad. Some people go without food for several days, even as long as a month. This is extremely dangerous.

Moderate fasting is helpful, but the stomach needs short intervals of rest on a daily basis. In my boyhood home "three square meals a day" were not considered sufficient. About midnight my mother would be back in the kitchen preparing a "snack" to tide us over until breakfast. What she usually came up with was a full-blown meal. No wonder I had recurring nightmares, and thought everyone woke up in the morning with a furry tongue. Stomachs in our family almost never had a chance to rest. Fortunately we learned better before any of our stomachs went on permanent strike.

It takes from three to five hours for the stomach to process food, so meals ought to be spaced about five hours apart. And nothing, absolutely *nothing*, should be eaten between meals. Even an apple or a handful of nuts will slow down the procedure and hold food in the stomach overtime. If you insist on keeping your digestive organs in perpetual motion, something is going to break down eventually.

Breakfast the most important meal

Actually, two meals a day are preferable to three, but such a regimen is difficult to follow with most of the world on a three-a-day schedule. At least we can heed the old adage to "Eat breakfast like a king, dinner like a prince, and supper like a pauper." Unfortunately, many of us have a tendency to get that order reversed. In fact, we are a nation of breakfast-skippers. If any of the three meals is to be left out, by all means it should be the evening meal.

"Breakfast" is just that—time to break a fast that began perhaps twelve or more hours before. Overnight is the longest time we go without food, so it shouldn't come as a surprise that breakfast is our most important meal. If we dash off to work without eating, or gulp down toast, jam, and coffee, we are automatically heading for trouble. By midmorning we run out of whatever steam we had upon arising, and become tired, fidgety, and generally hard to get along with. Many of the personnel problems at the office or factory may be the result of having so many breakfast-skippers under one roof.

A good breakfast gets the day started right. *From one third to one half of our day's total supply of essential nutrients should be provided by this early-morning meal.* Then the body has the necessary fuel to face the demands that lie ahead.

"But I'm just not hungry in the morning." Of course not. If you're an average American you stuff down a heavy meal at suppertime, and enjoy a little snack while watching television, as well. Try going without supper for a few days, and you'll begin to work up a good morning appetite. It may take a week or so to adjust, but don't give up. The habits of a lifetime don't drop away overnight.

When you think of abstemiousness, don't conjure up something dramatic like a Mohandas Gandhi-type fast. Instead, think in terms of a moderate intake of food on a regular day-to-day basis. The rewards of such a program are mental and moral vigor, keen perception, and the ability to arrive quickly at correct decisions. Try this way of living for a month or two and see whether it isn't something you'd like to adopt permanently.

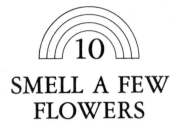

10

SMELL A FEW FLOWERS

BOB JOHNSON was a human dynamo. Warm and friendly, he possessed talents that opened doors of opportunity on every hand. And Bob was quick to walk through them, two or three at a time. He not only burned the candle at both ends but occasionally in the middle, as well. Long after most of the building was dark a light could be seen burning in his corner office on third floor. Bob was busy making his mark in the world.

And Bob did make quite a contribution to society before a heart attack cut him down at 43 years of age. Now, five years later, his name isn't mentioned very often. The world has a way of moving on. If only he had been a bit more careful about conserving his energy, he might have been around long enough to make an even greater contribution. And Susan wouldn't be struggling to be both mother and father to the three children Bob thought so much of.

Batteries aren't alone in their need for recharging. People too should "recharge" or "unwind" on a regular basis. A wise Providence has provided a built-in safety mechanism; we can go nonstop just so long before an overpowering urge to sleep overtakes us. Except for this wise arrangement, our many responsibilities would soon drive us into a state of physical and mental bankruptcy.

During sleep our muscles relax and our nervous system is relieved of the strain imposed upon it by the rigors of day-to-day living. This is the time when the body's repair-and-renewal program is at its peak.

Has that person in the mirror been looking a bit haggard lately? Good, sound sleep is one of the best beauty aids in the world. "According to some research, skin cells divide and make new cells about twice as fast while a person sleeps as they do when he's awake. In fact, next to proper nourishment, adequate sleep is probably the biggest factor in helping people look younger." [1]

Since approximately a third of a person's lifetime is spent in the Land of Nod, more attention should be given to this matter of sleep. Between the ages of 20 and 70 you will likely spend more than *fifteen full years in bed!* If you're one of those who never feels quite rested that statistic may be hard to believe.

How much sleep

Perhaps the most common question is "How much sleep do I need each night?" No one can provide a pat answer, as we each differ in our needs. Some people function perfectly well and feel rested on five hours' sleep a night; others just can't make it on less than nine or ten. The average seems to be about seven to eight hours. The main thing is not to worry about how much sleep you are supposed to have, but be concerned only about whether you get enough to keep from being tired. All sleep experts agree that the more *regular* the sleep hours, the better and more beneficial the sleep. Your body will provide you with trustworthy signals if you'll just pay attention.

Insomnia

Although seven minutes is the average time it takes for a person to drop off to sleep, a recent survey showed that more than half the adults in the United States are chronic insomniacs. Seeking relief, these people gobble down more than five hundred tons of sleeping pills annually.[2] In Great Britain sleeping pills account for 10 per cent of all prescriptions and even outsell aspirin.[3]

Chemically induced sleep may seem like a simple answer to a difficult problem, but those who seek their solution in a pill bottle are courting serious trouble. The most common danger with sleeping pills is habituation, which may even border on addiction. For some, this can lead to hard narcotic addiction. Habituation may result quickly, even when the pills are taken for only a short time.[4]

There is a better way to whip insomnia than by taking sleeping pills. If you enjoy spending money there are those ready to sell you water beds, vibrators, head clamps, special record albums, and fancy lights. But why not put your billfold or purse away and consider some safe and simple suggestions that will likely do the job?

How to whip insomnia

1. *Exercise more.* Increasing your activity during the day will make it much easier for you to fall asleep at night. Don't, however, do anything strenuous just before retiring. A brief, leisurely stroll is usually beneficial.

2. *Have a fixed time for going to bed.* We are creatures of habit, and dropping off to sleep should be a comfortable routine.

3. *Avoid late meals.* Don't eat anything during the hours just prior to retiring, and let the final meal of the day be light, perhaps fruit or soup.

4. *Don't nap in the evening.* Avoiding a nap too late in the day makes one more tired and ready for sleep.

5. *Take a warm bath.* A hot bath would prove stimulating and only compound the problem.

6. *Avoid stimulants.* Remember that coffee, tea, cola, and tobacco all tend to keep people awake.

7. *Practice deep breathing.* Breathe out through the mouth. Then draw in a deep breath through the nose, hold it for several seconds, and exhale through your nose as slowly as you can.

Wait a few seconds, and repeat the process.

8. *Learn to relax systematically.* Consciously think about completely relaxing each part of your body, starting at the top —the scalp, the forehead, the eyes, the ears, the mouth, the neck, the arms, the trunk, the legs, et cetera.

9. *Think of peaceful things.* Begin to unwind an hour or so before bedtime. Push away the worries and problems of the day, and occupy the mind with pleasant thoughts.

10. *Open the windows.* Treat your lungs to some fresh air. A cool room is more conducive to sleep than a warm one.

11. *Keep out unwanted light.* Pull the shades, or obtain a comfortable pair of eye covers.

12. *Seek quiet.* One may have to resort to ear plugs to cut out unwanted noise.

13. *Try counting sheep.* Don't laugh; it works. Dr. Richard Wyatt, of the National Institute of Mental Health says, "It's not so much the thinking about sheep, but doing a very repetitive and boring task. You know its outcome, so you can't get anxious or excited." Usually sleep eludes us because our mind is still actively milling over some problem; we need to slow down the mental processes.

I'm not particularly taken with sheep, so on those few nights each year when I have trouble falling asleep I just count, concentrating on the numbers themselves. I repeat each one very slowly and rarely do I ever reach fifty. If I occasionally get to one hundred I figure I'm not ready for sleep anyway, so I get up and do something useful.

Naps

I should have been born "south of the border" in siesta country, because I think the daytime nap is one of the greatest things ever invented. Why drag along at half speed, getting little accomplished, when a brief time out can recharge one's batteries. A sleep break is better than a coffee break anytime. If I can have just ten minutes of sleep I feel as fresh as if I were starting the day all over again. I keep a small blow-up pillow in my office closet, and if I feel too drowsy to accomplish much I lock the door and stretch out on the carpet. (Of course, if the general manager sees a copy of this book, I might find a slash cut in my blow-up pillow.)

Immediately after eating, a brief walk is preferable to a nap.

A dentist I am acquainted with has a built-in bunk in his office. If a patient fails to make an appearance or is unusually late, the dentist is on his bunk and asleep in no time. It's hard to develop an ulcer with that type of response.

In all fairness, I should point out that not all agree on the effectiveness of the ten-minute nap. My wife says that once she gets asleep nothing less than two hours will suffice, and I can testify she is ready to do battle with anyone who tries to wake her up.

Vacations

Occasionally we need to get completely away from it all for two or three weeks in a row. Don't let financial pressures keep you from taking your vacation. I once worked for an organization whose president insisted his men take their annual vacation period. He wasn't impressed by one old-timer who boasted that he had not had a vacation in thirteen years. Everyone believed him, because he was a most unpleasant, cantankerous person. A two-week rest might have helped to make him almost human.

That same president also insisted that one day a week every employee take his family somewhere beyond the reach of the telephone. He made it clear he wasn't trying to be magnanimous; adequately rested workers are better producers.

Remember, too, that a vacation is supposed to be restful. Trying to do all the scenic wonders of the nation in one 7,000-mile spasm is definitely not what the doctor ordered. Some people plan a vacation that is much harder than working, and they come back in worse condition than when they left. They need a week at home just to recuperate before they can face the job again. Sound familiar?

A proper vacation doesn't call for much highway travel. Don't try to jam too much into each 24-hour period; let the schedule be flexible and unhurried. Smell a few flowers, watch some sunsets, and get more sleep than usual. Luxuriate in the absence of alarm clocks, appointments, and deadlines. Much of your life is taken up with doing what other people want you to do when they want you to do it. Now, for a few days at least, you're the boss. Don't be a slave driver.

Keep it simple

Don't think that vacations have to be complicated to be enjoyable. A few years ago we rented a small house trailer in the upper peninsula of Michigan and parked it on the shore of Lake Superior. We never budged from that spot the entire time, and the most strenuous activity we engaged in was leisurely walking through the virgin hardwood forests nearby. We slept late, popped corn, played table games, and searched (unsuccessfully but happily) for agates on the beach. We felt a bit guilty about bringing our active teen-age daughter along on such a quiet, uneventful foray, but when it was all over she said, "Dad, that's the best vacation we've ever had. Please, let's do the same thing next year!"

And don't forget the possibilities for mini-vacations on those long weekends. Regardless of where you live, there are almost certainly a number of fascinating historical, educational, or inspirational spots within a few miles. Don't be forever reaching for the greener grass; do a little exploring right around home. It will pay rich dividends, and any change of pace helps make that next Monday morning a little bit brighter.

I've simply got to get off this subject. I find myself reaching impulsively for my suitcase, even though my vacation time is still months away.

Rest—one of nature's most effective remedies. If one is ill, a period of quiet rest can often bring complete restoration. If one is well, adequate periods of rest can help to maintain health.

---

[1] Shirley Motter Linde and Louis M. Savary, *The Sleep Book* (New York: Harper and Row, 1974), p. 81.

[2] Fred Kerner, *Stress and Your Heart* (New York: Hawthorne Books, 1961), pp. 95, 96.

[3] Shirley Motter Linde, *loc. cit.*

[4] *Ibid.*, p. 113.

"JANGLING GENTLY
AS YOU MOVE"

A FEW years ago I gazed upon one of the most awe-inspiring sights to be found in all the world, the great pyramid of Giza just outside Cairo, Egypt. Sometimes, places we have heard about from childhood prove to be disappointing in reality, but not so this man-made mountain jutting up out of the desert sands. Even stripped of its white-marble sheathing, it still speaks of the material glory of long-departed dynasties. Long departed, indeed. It is almost mind-boggling to consider that this same pyramid was a familiar sight to Moses, and no doubt also greatly impressed the parents of Jesus during their exile in Egypt.

Even today experts are unable to determine exactly how the pyramids were constructed without benefit of modern machinery. Although the specific techniques may remain a mystery, it is almost certain that a great deal of human muscle was involved.

Human muscle. Man-made mountains. Professor G. Stanley Hall put it well back in 1904 when he said that muscles "have built all the roads, cities, and machines in the world, written all the books, spoken all the words, and, in fact, done everything that man has accomplished with matter." That's a lot to say for a bit of tissue.

A push-button society

But today there seems to be a deliberate campaign to phase out muscle power. A good example comes to mind. As a teen-ager I had the responsibility (not a voluntary affair) to care for our home's heating system. Daily I shoveled coal from the bin into the furnace, filled the furnace water jackets, poked the fire regularly, and shook ashes down into a lower compartment. Since the national economy was in a depressed state, I also used a special sifting shovel to sort out pieces of coal that could be returned to the fire pot. Finally the ashes were dumped into a large tub, which I also had the privilege of carrying outside to empty.

Today I still have charge of the heating system, but my muscle output consists of turning the thermostat up in the fall and down again in the spring. Other members of the family regulate the temperature occasionally by gently moving their index finger an eighth of an inch in either direction.

Our grandparents didn't have to be concerned about exercise, not with pumping water, milking cows, feeding livestock, and hauling in firewood. And my own generation took it for granted that when young people wanted to go some place locally they walked or rode a bike. If a "heavy date" was involved, there was the possibility of negotiating for the family automobile. Now, unless Junior has his own personal sports car (with hi-jackers, headers, and mag wheels) by the time he's a junior in high school, he feels thoroughly deprived. Today's younger generation has been trained almost from birth to avoid exercise at all costs.

Ours is strictly a push-button society. About the only exercise many people today get is jumping to conclusions. Or walking from the TV set to the refrigerator during commercials. It used to be necessary to get out of the chair to change channels, but, of course, that problem has been solved by remote-control devices. Although most people still brush their teeth, even this modest bit of exercise is endangered by the inroads of the electric toothbrush.

Designed for action

The craze for labor-saving gadgets might be taken as a sign the human muscular system is extremely delicate and needs continual babying. Such is most assuredly not the case. Actually, the human body is designed to thrive on usage.

Man has about 600 skeletal muscles made up of more than 6 billion muscle fibers. He is able to perform tasks because these miraculous little fibers are capable of contracting and relaxing, deriving their energy from the food we eat. Although tiny, about the size of a human hair, each muscle fiber can support 1,000 times its own weight. Delicate? Hardly.

And this wonderful muscular system is orchestrated to perform feats so intricate as to be almost beyond comprehension. Consider something as "simple" as a baseball pitcher delivering his fast ball. Here's how a Professor Harvey described the action back in 1931:

"When a baseball pitcher stands on his feet and throws a ball from his hand, he uses parts of almost every muscle in the body—some in the legs and trunk to produce and hold the desired position and others in the arms and hands to throw the ball. When he wants more force (strength or tension) he calls on a few thousand more motor units that he has not been using in pitching slower balls or he increases the rate with which those already used were bombarded with nerve impulses. Some of the extra force is furnished by arm muscles, but much of it comes from legs and trunk. He can combine any part of each with any part of all the others. As the pitcher goes through the successive stages of his pitching motion, the parts and combinations change in progressive order: now he winds up—then the right leg muscles throw him suddenly forward with full force—then the right shoulder muscles swing his right arm, ending with a final spasm of all the power of the pectorals as the arm muscles gripping the ball through their finger tendons make the throw. Incurve, outcurve, or drop curve?—the arm muscles do it in the last tiny fragment of a second. Then they stop suddenly. The pitcher has let go of the ball; it has just the right speed and just the right spin on it for sixty feet away it curves over the inner corner of the plate exactly where the catcher signaled him to put it. Seconds are much too long as a time measure in the game. The pitcher can shift his muscle action forty times a second. The delivery of no two pitchers is alike; each has worked up his own style. It is the result of particular combinations of muscle fibers." [1]

Obviously the human body was designed to be highly active, and we needn't be surprised if our modern aversion to movement produces difficulties. The mechanical equipment around your house loses a little ground every time you use it, but every time your body is exercised it actually gains. Muscles don't care anything about the machine age; they just keep on begging to be used.

"Begging to be used." If you have a sedentary job and have been cheating on your exercise, you know precisely what I'm talking about. More than once you have found it almost impossible to concentrate on your paper work because your leg muscles were screaming for attention. Such physical distress is almost painful. You probably had to get up and move around a bit before you could resume your work.

Continually ignoring the pleas of unused muscles finally brings on a state of general unfitness. You know the signs: getting completely out of breath with every little exertion, habitually appearing nervous and tense, and feeling tired and dragged out almost every waking hour. Not a very flattering description, but unfortunately it characterizes the average man or woman in this country today.

The price of inactivity

Since action is a law of our very being, inaction is a fruitful cause of disease. Eventually we have to pay the piper. The under-exercised person may look all right, and at the moment there might not be very much wrong with him. On the other hand, there isn't very much right about him, either. Trouble is on the way; it just hasn't arrived yet. Dr. Hans Krause has coined a special word to describe the broad spectrum of physical and mental derangements that stem from inactivity. He calls them *hypokinetic* diseases, i.e., diseases "caused by insufficient motion."

Employers are just beginning to realize that their employees' flabbiness hurts—right in the pocketbook. Loss of production as a result of premature death and illness in the United States alone amounts to billions of dollars per year. A healthy worker contributes more when he's on the job and loses less time from the job.

Many business concerns are doing something constructive about the problem. Some provide recreational facilities for off-hour use. Others are laying out special exercise trails through nearby wooded areas. One organization I visited has outfitted a spare room with two or three treadmills. Each employee knows that if at any time during the working day those muscles are "clamoring to be used," he or she is welcome to take a few brief strides on a treadmill. No one need feel guilty, as everyone stands to gain.

Just how bad is the picture? Dr. Kenneth H. Cooper, of aerobics fame, claims that "only one American in five can be considered truly fit." It isn't a problem restricted to those more than 40 years of age. During World War II draft boards were shocked to learn that a large percentage of young recruits couldn't begin to pass the necessary physicals. More recently, Dr. Cortez P. Enloe, Jr., points out:

"According to unpublished data, among the thousands of healthy young men to have been killed in the Indochina war and come to autopsy, pathologists have discovered well-developed lesions of atherosclerosis in more than fifty out of every hundred soldiers examined." [2]

Lest we be accused of male chauvinism, may we hasten to point out that women are not excluded from this state of general unfitness. The average housewife is quick to proclaim, "Don't worry about any lack of exercise on my part. I run up and down stairs all day." But the electronic gadgets surrounding today's housewife have taken over many of the former tasks calling for muscle involvement. Supplemental exercise is called for, as the heart-attack rate in women is steadily inching upward.

Benefits

Although the liabilities connected with a lack of exercise are serious, the benefits to be derived from adequate exercise are also impressive. Participants about to join an adult physical-fitness program carried on by the YMCA gave "continual fatigue" as their number one complaint. Strangely enough, the cure for this particular kind of tiredness is not rest, but *more* activity. But overcoming fatigue was only one benefit realized. Those involved in the exercise program over a period of time reported a gradual lessening of such complaints as digestive upsets, heartburn, acid stomach, diabetic tendency, constipation, headaches, fat, hemorrhoids, heart thumping, chest pain, abdominal pain, painful feet, eye watering, sinus trouble, and swollen joints.[3]

It is important that we understand the greatest possible good to come from a proper exercise regimen. Since 53 per cent of all deaths in the United States result from diseases of the heart and blood vessels, we would naturally look in that direction.

Oxygen is the key

Every cell in the body is dependent upon life-giving oxygen. Any activity we engage in requires energy, and this energy is produced when our food is burned by oxidation. We can go for weeks without food, about eleven days without drink, but hardly a dozen minutes without oxygen. Since it is the blood that carries this vital substance throughout the body, anything that improves circulation is going to be highly beneficial. Exercise does just that. Although he is not a physiologist, the ageless baseball-player Satchel Paige was batting a thousand when he urged concerning exercise, "Keep the juices flowing by jangling gently as you move."

Here's how exercise affects the circulatory system. The tiniest blood vessels, the capillaries, penetrate into muscles, spinal cord, brain, lungs, nerves, and organs in general. They are responsible for irrigating the tissues of the entire body. When a person is at rest only a few of these capillaries will be open, but when a muscle is being exercised perhaps 50 times as many will open up. It is believed that through consistent exercise, even the number of capillaries is increased.

During extreme exercise, the rate of blood flow through a muscle may increase as much as 15- to 20-fold. Obviously the body tissues are going to be thoroughly irrigated by this kind of circulation.

The heart is a most amazing and durable muscle. It faithfully beats about 200,000 times each day, pumping more than 2,000 gallons of blood! A physically inactive person may have a resting heart rate of 80 beats per minute. By systematic and regular exercise, the heart can supply in 60 beats what previously took 80 or more. Just figure it out. That means a saving of 28,000 heart beats each day. No wonder twice as many inactive people have heart attacks as do those who are physically active. If a heart is in good condition it can double or even triple its output when necessary without undue strain.

The benefits to the human body to be derived from adequate exercise are invaluable. Let's take a brief look at them again.

Exercise:

1. Increases circulation
2. Assists the heart and protects against premature heart disease
3. Increases the supply of oxygen to the body
4. Aids digestion
5. Relaxes the nerves and balances the emotions
6. Increases resistance to disease
7. Reduces fatigue
8. Strengthens muscles, bones, and ligaments
9. Beautifies the figure and complexion
10. Sharpens the mental powers
11. Enhances poise and agility
12. Protects against sudden stress, either physical or emotional

13. Improves glandular function
14. Strengthens motivation, confidence, and will power
15. Improves posture
16. Helps induce sound sleep

No matter how rich you are, you can't buy benefits like these at any price. No matter how poor you are, you can enjoy these benefits by merely giving a few minutes each day to a consistent, sensible exercise program.

What type of exercise?

When it comes to general fitness, looks can be deceiving. We might easily suppose that the weight lifter with the Atlas-like body represents the very epitome of good health, but the truth is that those bulging biceps may be hiding a flabby heart muscle ready to give up at any moment. Isometric exercises and calisthenics are all right, but they cannot accomplish the all-important task of building up your heart and lungs. This calls for a different approach.

Enthusiasts will argue avidly that their particular exercise program is best, but actually there are numerous possibilities. Pick a regimen that is tailor-made for you. The following suggestions may help in making such a selection.

First of all, find something you are going to enjoy. If you hate every minute of your program it isn't going to last. As with most crash diets, it will probably fade away after a week or so. Then you will be right back with your guilty conscience. Find something you like to do, something that will remain a permanent part of your life-style month after month and year after year.

Keep it simple. Anything that is highly complicated also tends to dampen enthusiasm.

It doesn't have to be expensive. There are gadgets galore on the market, and some of them no doubt are well designed, but you can do just as well for pennies.

There are certain advantages to selecting an exercise that can be carried on in all kinds of weather. The fewer excuses you have to skip a day, the better.

Your exercise program should be something you can do on a daily basis, or at least three times a week. The worst thing is to sit around all week and then try to act like an Olympic champion on Sunday. Ambulance drivers are kept busy with calls from people like that.

Remember, too, the basic principle of moderation that should govern our entire approach to health. Drs. Friedman and Rosenman have given good advice in their book, *Type A Behavior and Your Heart:*

"Persons of all ages, if they do not suffer already from crippling coronary heart disease, should indulge in as much moderate physical activity as they possibly can. Certainly at least one hour a day and preferably more time should be spent in moving your legs and arms.

"By moderate physical activity, we mean any form of exercise whose execution does not cause panting, excessive acceleration of your heartbeat (that is, above 120 beats per minute), or leave you unduly fatigued. . . .

"Persons over thirty-five years of age should not indulge in severe forms of exercise, regardless of how long and how often they indulged in such exercises previously, or how healthy they may think that they are, unless they have undergone an electrocardiographic checkup while walking or jogging on a treadmill at top speed of five miles per hour. . . . The ordinary electrocardiogram taken as you lie supine on a cot just won't do." [4]

There are so many legitimate forms of exercise available to the average person, it would be impossible to list them all. We will mention only a few. No matter what your age, ability, or interest, with a little bit of research you should be able to find an exercise program perfectly tailored to your individual needs.

Swimming

Swimming has long been recognized as one of the best exercises. This form of activity can easily be adapted to a wide range of individual responses, from the youngest to the eldest, from the least fit to the trained athlete. Purposeful swimming properly involves the heart and the lungs. The entire cardio-vascular system is strengthened and toned.

Walking

The most popular form of exercise in the United States for both men and women is walking. Dr. Paul Dudley White said, "It is the easiest exercise for most individuals, one that can be done without equipment except good shoes, in almost any terrain and weather, and into very old age. . . . The best way to keep fit is to walk and walk and walk."

There is some basis of fact for the old saying, "I have two doctors, my left leg and my right." The human muscular system acts as an auxiliary blood pump, thus saving the heart from extra exertion. The leg muscles are especially important, since they are the largest and most powerful in the body. When in action, they help squeeze the blood back toward the heart, but, of course, they have to be used vigorously to be most effective.

When you are out for exercise don't meander down the street peering into shop windows. We are talking about striding, moving out at a brisk pace with head up and shoulders back. You will know when you have "hit your stride," as each person has a gait that feels just right for him. And don't be surprised if after a few blocks you can't even remember the problems you were carrying when you first started out.

Although violent exercise of any kind immediately after a meal is injurious, a brief walk will prove to be highly beneficial. Five minutes of striding will promote digestion and prove better than a nap.

Gardening

Any exercise outdoors has a built-in bonus, as the lungs are nourished by the fresh air. Not only does serious gardening provide a good workout but getting that close to nature also does something for the soul. Those tomatoes from your own vine are redder, juicier, tastier—and much, much cheaper.

Nothing like getting your exercise and helping to balance the family food budget at the same time.

Jumping rope

I can't resist putting in a commercial for my own personal exercise program. My equipment was purchased for pennies— a nine-foot length of nylon rope, suitable for jumping. In good weather I can be in the open air; in bad weather there is no problem jumping indoors.

" 'For producing the greatest fitness in the least amount of time,' says Dr. Kaare Rodahl, eminent head of the Institute of Work Physiology in Oslo, Norway, 'nothing surpasses the simple jump rope.' " [5] This form of conditioning is included in training programs at West Point and was used by a number of the astronauts.

Jumping rope has certain advantages over jogging. For one thing, the rhythmic turning of the rope exercises more of the upper body than jogging does. And studies at Arizona State University comparing jumping and jogging indicated that, for improving cardiovascular efficiency, ten minutes with the rope is equal to thirty on the road.

Some years ago Dr. Rodahl, then director of research at Lankenav Hospital in Philadelphia, decided to see whether jumping rope could counteract the midafternoon fatigue of his staff members, women whose ages were between 19 and 24. They jumped rope for five minutes a day, during the lunch hour, five days a week. In one month, their physical-work capacity increased by an average of 25 per cent!

Just writing on this topic got me highly inspired. I grabbed my trusty rope, always close at hand, and dashed into the hall outside my office for a few quick turns. The timing was unfortunate, for the night watchman was just making his rounds on third floor. I could still see his startled countenance as he turned the hall corner, and I hoped he wasn't heading for the nearest telephone. This is just one of the many hazards one faces in attempting to keep fit in a society dedicated to remaining unfit.

Limbering up

Another good practice is limbering up for the day. I have developed my own simple set of calisthenics to loosen up all major body joints. The stress is on simplicity, so that the routine doesn't become a burden. It takes only three or four minutes, and everything is done from a standing or squatting position. If the routine calls for lying on one's back, doing push-ups, et cetera, things begin to get complicated. A few faithful souls will go through such a procedure every morning, but most will soon simply forget the whole thing.

While your routine should be simple, it must be consistent. We have "instant" soup, "instant" cereal, and "instant" almost everything, but there is no such things as an "instant" exercise program. The only possible way of gaining circulatory fitness is by a *systematic* method of exercise. It must become as much a part of your life-style as eating or sleeping.

Then throw in a little extra activity for good measure. Shun the elevator and take the stairs. Deliberately leave your car at the far end of the parking lot when visiting the shopping center. If you are fortunate enough to live within a reasonable walking distance from your work, by all means walk.

A serious warning

A special warning is in order for anyone who has suffered a heart attack or who suspects he may have coronary difficulties. Again, may we urge readers to check on their true condition, particularly if over the age of 40, by taking a carefully controlled treadmill stress test. Listen to Drs. Friedman and Rosenman once again:

"We wish to emphasize that coronary arteries aren't heart muscles—they don't get 'accustomed' to regular exercise even if it is severe. No one ever made a diseased coronary artery more 'physically fit.' " [6]

You probably have a scar somewhere on an arm or leg. Has it become smaller through the years because of exercising that limb? A diseased coronary artery is considered diseased because of the obstructing scars it bears, and such arteries become dangerous only when they deteriorate and rupture. The abovementioned specialists continue:

"As a coronary patient, your danger does not lie in the ability of your heart muscle to contract well or to extract oxygen from the blood passing through it. Your only danger lies in the tough, stone-containing scars that are obliterating the interior portions of your coronary arteries. And if you were to ascend and descend the Pyramid of Cheops at Giza a dozen times a day at jogging speed for a decade, you still would not widen or open any of your coronary vessels where they had been severely narrowed or entirely closed. You would succeed only in breaking your neck or dying instantaneously of a cardiac arrhythmia." [7]

Invalids

Many who are invalids could be restored to health by a well-planned exercise program. They are slowly dying of indolence. Proper exercise would bring into use those enfeebled muscles, enliven the stagnant blood in the system, and arouse a sluggish liver to perform its necessary work. A strengthening of the muscles of respiration would facilitate the rapid flow of air in and out of the lungs, and result in much good.

Obesity

We are going to talk later about the problem of overweight, but it would be wrong not to mention it here, because exercise is a big factor in whipping that particular problem. Listen carefully to Dr. Jean Mayer of Harvard University, one of the most outstanding nutritionists in the nation today:

"Whether we are obese or not still depends on the relationship between the amount of food we eat and the energy we use. Actually, the *major* factor is not hormones or heredity or glucoreceptors, but physical inactivity. . . . If you are very inactive, you eat a certain amount. If your activity goes up, we find that your food intake tends to go *down* a little bit. It certainly doesn't increase. It increases only when your activity is decidedly greater. We can get people to lose weight simply by exercising them more. . . . We have had programs in which we have reduced hundreds of children without touching their food intake, simply by increasing their physical activity." [8]

Did you catch that lovely phrase?—"without touching their food intake." It is quite possible that you can eat what you want, within reason, and still keep your weight where it ought to be if you will only exercise properly. Isn't that a pretty good incentive, along with all the other wonderful benefits that accrue to the active person? It surely has to be worth a try.

Hopefully we have said enough to prod your conscience if you are guilty of skimping on your exercise. Few things will pay as many dividends as being faithful in this area. Dr. Thomas Cureton has summed it up this way: "It is quite probable that the fountain of youth for middle-aged people will be found in the wise use of leisure time to maintain their physical fitness." [9]

Escape once and for all from the fatigue and boredom of today's sedentary way of life. Wake up, move out, and really live!

[1] Arthur H. Steinhaus, *Toward an Understanding of Health and Physical Education* (Dubuque, Iowa: Wm. C. Brown Co., Publishers, 1963), p. 15.

[2] Cortez P. Enloe, Jr., M.D., "Progress and Patience," *Nutrition Today*, May/June, 1971, p. 14.

[3] Thomas K. Cureton, Ph.D., F.A.C.S.M., *The Physiological Effects of Exercise Programs on Adults* (Springfield, Ill.: Charles C. Thomas, Publisher, 1969), pp. 8, 9.

[4] From *Type A Behavior and Your Heart*, by Meyer Friedman, M.D., and Ray H. Rosenman, M.D. Copyright © 1974 by Meyer Friedman. Reprinted by permission of Alfred A. Knopf, Inc. In U.K. and Europe rights are held by Wildwood House, Ltd., London. Reprinted by permission. Pp. 156, 157.

[5] Curtis Mitchell, "Hop, Skip and Jump to Health," *Reader's Digest*, May, 1974, pp. 37-42.

[6] Friedman and Rosenman, *op. cit.*, p. 158.

[7] *Ibid.*, p. 255.

[8] Jean Mayer, Ph.D., interviewed by Marjorie Baldwin, M.D., "The Scoop—In a Nutshell," Obesity, *Life and Health* Supplement, 1974, p. 13.

[9] Cureton, *op. cit.*, p. 16.

NATURE'S NEEDFUL NECTAR

THE FIRST astronauts to escape the bonds of gravitation and soar on out into space looked back on an incredibly beautiful sight—Planet Earth. The other planets appear to be desolate wastelands, wracked with terrifying extremes of searing heat and numbing cold. But Earth is a unique jewel hung in the vastness of space; a delicate blue orb traced with swirling white cloud patterns.

The "blue planet" derives its pleasing color from the seas and oceans that cover nearly four fifths of its surface. Without these great bodies of water our world could not support human life. Yet that water is a limited and destructible commodity. While we learn how to use it, we should also learn how to preserve it.

Few are aware of the significant role water plays in our very existence. From 50 to 65 per cent of the human body is water, depending on one's size and general make-up. Muscles are 75 per cent water, and even bones are more than 20 per cent water. Every one of our 100 million cells requires fluid. Every chemical and electrical reaction of the body takes place in a liquid medium. Every time you swallow, lift a box, scratch your back, swing a tennis racket, or write a letter, you use water.

Water power

For decades ambitious climbing teams from all over the world assaulted the rocky flanks of the world's highest peak, Mount Everest. None lacked in courage and dedication, and many lives were lost in those attempts, but the great stone fortress seemed impregnable. Then came the electrifying news that Sir Edmund Hillary and Tenzing Norgay had planted their flags on the very rooftop of the world.

Do you know why those two men succeeded where all others had failed? According to the physician attending the winning team, plain water made the difference. The members of the teams that failed were drinking only about two glasses of water a day, and this resulted in numbing exhaustion. Hillary and Norgay forced themselves to drink regularly twelve glasses of water a day. You may not have any mountains to climb, but if even a modest-sized molehill looks impossible by midafternoon, it may be you just aren't drinking enough water.

Use it on the inside

Years ago even feverish patients were often denied an adequate supply of life-giving water. Now we know that everyone ought to drink copious amounts of this vital fluid each day. How much? Of course, needs vary with the weather and the type of activity one is engaged in. On a hot day two or more quarts of fluid may be lost through the lungs and skin. Obviously our water intake ought to be stepped up accordingly on such a day.

On the average we should be certain to drink a minimum of six glasses of water daily, and eight would be even better. The kidneys act as a wonderful filtering system, but they can do a good job only if they have an adequate supply of water. Plan to drink two glasses of water upon rising in the morning, two glasses about halfway between breakfast and lunch, and two more glasses about mid-afternoon.

Perhaps you noticed we didn't suggest drinking anything with your meals. There is a very good reason for this. If you drink with your meals, the liquid not only diminishes the flow of saliva but also dilutes the stomach acids needed to process your food. Before the stomach can actually get at its task, it must first absorb the water that has been introduced. Once again: for optimum health, do not wash down your food. If you drink plenty of water between meals, the desire for it at mealtime will not be so great.

It is wise to stay completely away from iced drinks. They arrest digestion until the system has imparted sufficient warmth to the stomach to enable it to take up its work once again. If the cooler in the hallway is set at too low a temperature obtain a glass and drink from the tap.

The soda pop craze

No drink has ever been devised that even approaches the perfection of water—but people keep trying. They shun nature's offering and turn to coffee, tea, hot chocolate, or fruit-flavored ades. The national thirst for soda pop has reached alarming proportions.

In 1971 America's soft-drink bill was a staggering 5 billion dollars! That means the average citizen downed some 390 bottles, and consumption has gone up considerably since that time. Young people in grades 7 to 12 list soda pop as their "most liked" food.

With a sugar content ranging from 10 to 15 per cent, soft drinks hardly rate as food at all. The 100 calories in an ordinary 8-ounce bottle contain very few nutrients; they are largely "empty" calories. And even worse, these soft drinks and fruit ades crowd out of the diet such protective foods as milk, fruit, and fruit juices. Especially in children this poses a serious nutritional problem.* That is in addition to the damage the sugar does to their teeth.

Use it on the outside

The value of water for bathing is a comparatively new concept. Years ago exposing so much of one's anatomy to a good wetting was considered not only unnecessary but downright dangerous. Even Europe's palaces contained no bathrooms, and the only tub at Versailles was finally turned into a fountain because no one used it. Perfume was worn not so much to introduce delightful new odors as to mask unpleasant ones. At least; it made socializing bearable.

Regular bathing is not only a fine social custom, it is absolutely essential to good health. The skin is a most useful organ when it comes to giving off bodily impurities, but if the skin is not cleansed, and the clothing as well, these impurities may be reabsorbed. The sebaceous glands are continually pouring their oily secretions upon the skin, and if these are not removed each day the pores become clogged and form fertile culture for growing bacteria.

Anyone who has become accustomed to a daily bath knows that such a practice is anything but a chore. A hot or cold bath is exhilarating, and when a person feels clean and refreshed he faces the world with a greater degree of confidence and vitality.

For that glowing feeling

Perhaps the best time of the day for a bath is early in the morning. If you want something really invigorating to get you off to a supercharged start, try this routine:

1. In a comfortably warm room, probably your bathroom, fill a basin with tepid or slightly warm water.

2. Dip a rough washcloth (or you can buy a regular friction mitt at a drugstore) into the water and then wring it nearly dry.

3. Rub a portion of your body briskly until the skin is pink or until you feel a nice warm glow.

4. Dry that part with a warm towel, and then continue accordingly until the entire body has been rubbed down.

The remarkable effect of this routine is not merely psychological. The brisk rubbing improves circulation and sends blood speeding along more freely through your blood vessels. Every organ of the body is benefited, and you naturally feel better.

Some devotees of the friction rub say that the best effects are obtained when cooler or even ice water is used. More hardy readers may want to check this out personally.

Water's medicinal attributes

Don't overlook plain water as an effective remedy. People who drink two glasses of warm or hot water upon arising are not likely to have to spend money on laxatives.

A tepid or neutral bath is a wonderful soother of the nerves, and also a good cure for insomnia.

Think of all the germ-laden materials you handle daily; money, for example. Frequently washing the hands, particularly before meals, is a good safeguard against disease.

The heating compress

The next time Junior has a sore throat have your physician arrange for a throat culture in order to detect a potentially serious beta-strep infection. If the sore throat is not a severe problem try this instead of heading for the drugstore to purchase something that tastes great and accomplishes little. Just at bedtime, wring a handkerchief or strip of thin cloth out of ice water and place around the child's neck. (If he's going to protest, it will be at this point. Don't weaken.) Then cover the cold, wet cloth with a warm, dry strip of wool flannel large enough to cover the neck thoroughly (a large wool sock can substitute if necessary), and pin in place. Make sure all the damp cloth is covered. In the morning remove the compress, wipe the neck with a cloth rinsed in tepid water, and pat dry with a warm towel. More often than not, the soreness will be completely gone.

This highly effective treatment was not picked up from a witch doctor, but has a simple physiological explanation behind it. Soon after being covered with the flannel, the cold, wet cloth begins to warm up. It finally becomes quite warm and continues to heat the skin until it dries itself out. Throughout the night it has drawn to the affected area a rich supply of blood, which brings disease-fighting properties.

Gargling hot water with a dash of salt is also helpful. In any case, nature's way is superior to indiscriminate drugging. If a sore throat persists in spite of such simple treatments, then one should see a physician.

There is an entire system of treating various ailments with hot and cold water, known as *hydrotherapy*. It is beyond the scope of this small volume to go into greater detail, but the reader may wish to investigate further on his own.

Our polluted waters

Have you ever thought about the wonder of merely turning a tap in your home and having instantly available cool drinkable water? Even today this isn't possible every place in the world. I lived for some time in a country where the water lines and the sewer lines were reportedly a bit interconnected. The only safe course was to carefully boil every drop of water that came from the tap, before drinking. Servants were normally responsible for maintaining the supply of drinking water. Following the boiling process, the water was poured into large clay pots where it cooled for drinking. Unfortunately, many servants were not really sold on the germ theory. Anyone with common sense could hold a glass of tap water up to the light and see it was clear, with nothing wriggling or swimming around. The foreigners were obviously a bit odd, and what they didn't know wouldn't hurt them.

I'm sure some of the water went directly from the tap right into the clay pots without benefit of boiling. And what I didn't know did hurt me. I not only endured the misery of amebic dysentery but suffered from typhoid fever as well. Back in the United States it seemed a minor miracle to hold a drinking glass directly under a water tap without any concern.

I hope we never lose this minor miracle. According to recent reports, much of our drinking water is now suspect because of inadequate treatment systems and our drawing of water from polluted sources. We need to do whatever is necessary to ensure a safe supply of drinking water.

Just the other day I ran across a map indicating the location of a fresh-water spring near my own home. A note said it is regularly inspected by the county health department. When time permits, I'm going to check it out.

Whether for internal or external use, water is one of man's most priceless possessions. Don't waste it; treat it like the precious commodity it really is.

---

* Lydia Sonnenberg, "The Soda Pop Craze," *Life and Health*, August, 1973, pp. 31-33.

WEEVILS ARE SMARTER
THAN PEOPLE

IN PRACTICING dentistry my father is often dismayed by what he finds in the mouths of even very young patients. Boys and girls not yet old enough to enter school already suffer rampant tooth decay. And these are not youngsters from poverty-stricken homes, but those whose parents have adequate funds to supply the necessities of life. Malnourishment in the midst of plenty; how strange.

My dad's answer to this problem, although drastic, has often proved effective. It goes something like this:

"Mrs. Jones, your son's mouth is in a rather deplorable condition."

"Well, I was afraid that might be the case."

"There are numerous cavities to be filled, and a couple of teeth may even have to be removed. I have an idea. How would you like to adopt a routine that would keep your son's teeth strong and healthy?"

"That would certainly be wonderful. What would we have to do?"

"Do you have a dog?" (Many families with small children have a pet dog. A cat will serve the purpose, as well.)

"Why yes, we have a small poodle. Why?"

"Actually it's very simple. Tomorrow begin feeding

your dog whatever you have been feeding your son, and let your son eat the commercial dog food you've been buying for the poodle. In a few months all the holes will be in the dog's teeth, and your son will be in great shape."

Of course, this is all for the shock value. Many parents get the point and begin thinking seriously about the family diet. They have seen the analysis of nutrients listed on the side of the dog food can, and suddenly they realize they have been more concerned about their pet's physical welfare than that of their own children.

It isn't only dogs and cats that fare so well. The average farmer is more concerned about what he feeds his hogs than some housewives are about what they place on the dinner table. It's time we did some soul searching about this matter of proper nutrition.

You are what you eat

If anyone ever tells you you're not the man, or woman, you used to be, don't argue with them; they're absolutely right. Previously we stated that the brain cells you were born with are the only ones you'll ever have, so you should take good care of them. On the other hand, nearly all the other cells in your body are continually changing. Each day millions of these cells are dying and being disposed of, while other millions of brand-new cells are taking their place. So, you see, the "you" of today, physically speaking, is not the "you" of ten years ago. A rather strange thought, isn't it?

This matter is more than just interesting. New cells have to come from somewhere; they have to be made of something. The fact is that these new cells are built up from the food we consume each day. Right away you can begin to see why a proper diet is so vital. It is no more possible to build a strong body with poor food than to build a strong house with termite-ridden lumber. The old adage "you are what you eat" is essentially true.

Doctors George Mann and Frederick Stare of the Harvard School of Public Health have put it plainly: *"In our opinion, nutrition is the most important single environmental factor affecting health."* In his book *You're the Doctor*, Dr. Victor G. Heiser, public health administration consultant, has added, "Your diet, what you eat, largely influences the rate at which your organism ages, and consequently the duration of your life."

When we talk about diet we are discussing one of the most important subjects we could possibly consider, so let us give it careful attention.

What constitutes a good diet?

As never before in history, people are concerned about their health. Many seem ready and even anxious to take whatever steps are necessary to feel fit and live longer. Unfortunately a small army of profiteers stands ready to take advantage of the situation. With the cash register ringing in their ears, they lead the gullible down any path promising a quick profit. Today the uninformed seeker of health may not only be wasting his money but actually may be purchasing poor health in place of good. Let's take a brief look at some of the booby traps along the way.

Faddist diets

If a person is searching for some far-out diet, he won't have to look long. There is a veritable smorgasbord of offerings: the high protein-low carbohydrate diet, the high carbohydrate-low protein diet, the "eat your way to thinness" diet, the grapefruit diet, the watermelon diet, the skimmed milk and banana diet, the liquid formula diet, the yogurt diet, the vinegar-kelp-lecithin-B_6 diet, the Zen macrobiotic diet, and others. Some of these fad routines are relatively harmless nonsense; others are positively dangerous. A few, like the Zen macrobiotic diet, if followed religiously over a period of time can result in death. The only intelligent course is to learn what proper nutrition is all about and put it into actual practice.

Organic foods

Many people today drive extra miles and spend extra money for foods labeled "organic." Unless you have more time and money than you know what to do with, don't concern yourself with this popular fad. For one thing, although "about 3 per cent of the American food supply is marketed as organically grown, *only a fraction of 1 per cent of our agricultural land is under organic cultivation.*" [1] This fact alone ought to cause one to tighten his hold on his billfold. But there is more.

A plant product is, by definition, made up of certain nutrients. And these nutrients are not there merely for human benefit, but are needed by the plant itself for growth and metabolism. For instance, a grapefruit cell needs more vitamin C than does a carrot cell. A carrot cell, on the other hand, needs more provitamin A than that of a grapefruit cell. Each kind of cell needs the minimum nutrients its structure calls for in order to exist at all. It simply is not true that a beautiful-looking apple may have no food value. If the soil had enough nutrients to produce an apple at all, that apple is going to be good for food—and it doesn't make any difference whether the tree was fertilized with decomposed plant or animal material or a commercial fertilizer, provided it gets enough of what it needs.

Is there no reason, then, for taking care of our soil? Yes, there is. Suppose we have two farmers raising wheat. One fertilizes his land, rotates his crops, and allows his field to lie fallow occasionally. The other does nothing but plant and reap. At harvesttime, the first farmer is going to be rewarded with many *more* bushels of wheat to the acre.

But were we to grind grain from each man's crop and bake two loaves of bread, both loaves would be nutritious. Even a nutritionist would not be able to determine which loaf originated from which field.

The conclusion? Variations in the nutritive value of foods grown on different soils are of little import as far as diet is concerned.[2] Your food dollar can be better spent than on so-called organic foods.

Massive vitamin doses

If you observe someone popping pills throughout the day, don't automatically assume they're hooked on drugs. It's quite possible they're downing large amounts of vitamin C in an effort to fend off a cold, or gobbling vitamin E tablets hoping to stave off old age. But before you join them, consider a few pertinent facts.

The seven constituents of food are as follows (vitamins being only a part):

1. *Proteins* are to build and repair body tissue. Some protein foods are meat, eggs, milk, cheese, peanut butter, peas, and beans. From 10 to 15 per cent of our calories should be protein.

2. *Carbohydrates* provide energy for the body. They are found in grain products, sweets, fruits, and vegetables. From 60 to 70 per cent of our calories should be carbohydrate.

3. *Fats* also contribute energy and help us to absorb certain fat-soluble vitamins.

4. *Vitamins* are involved in the regulation of body processes. Without them neither energy nor tissue can be produced by the body.

5. *Minerals* form healthy bones and teeth, and help nerves and muscles react normally.

6. *Cellulose* supplies the bulk needed for maintaining good muscular tone in the intestinal tract.

7. *Water* we have already considered in detail in another chapter.

Since vitamins and minerals are absolutely essential for bodily functions, some assume that the more they take the healthier they are bound to be. But there is danger in tampering too drastically with bodily chemistry. Vitamins, for instance, are so potent that they are measured in thousandths of a gram—that is, one one-thousandth of one quarter of a teaspoonful!

A good example of this potency is vitamin B_{12}. Just one one-millionth of a gram each day is all that is needed to perfectly regulate some of your most important and delicate bodily functions. Do you see how there could be danger in gulping down handfuls of these powerful substances? An excess of one vitamin may directly oppose the vital function of another. There is even the possibility of toxic (poisonous) reaction.

"Experiences during the last few years . . . show how urgent the need is for the public as well as scientists to understand the concept that all nutrients are only safe or useful to the body within limited quantitative range. . . . Whether or not they are useful or essential; they are all harmful if consumed in excessive quantities."[3]

While we're at it, we would also like to assure you that it doesn't make any difference whether vitamins are synthetic (manufactured) or natural (extracted from foods). Inside the body they react the same way.

Remember that someone is always busy inventing new ways to part you and your money. I have in hand a catalog that just came through the mail. According to the company that puts it out, the only way I can hope to survive (let alone be healthy) is to take large quantities of everything they advertise. And that isn't easy. They start on page one with vitamins A, B, C, D, and then some. Moving into the mining business they offer everything from iron to zinc. From there on it gets more exotic. Every day I should be sure to get my quota of sea salt, lecithin, linseed oil, kelp, bone meal, dolomite, rose hips, and ginseng. I may have to give up my job just to be able to keep up with the ordering and ingesting.

Why not spend your money on some nice fresh fruit? Good health is not to be found in a handbag full of pill bottles. According to the American Dietetic Association:

"Healthy individuals do not need vitamin, mineral, and dietary supplements if an adequate diet is consumed. A varied diet selected from the basic food groups will provide an adequate diet for optimal health." [4]

An adequate diet

Providing your family with an adequate, well-balanced diet is not as complicated as you might suppose. With a bit of know-how and some judicious shopping, such a diet can be obtained quite easily from your local supermarket. A good rule is to choose each day from the—

Four basic food groups:

1. Protein group; 2 or more servings.
   Beans, peas, lentils, nuts, peanut butter, cheese, eggs, and meat analogs. (We'll explain later what "meat analogs" are and how they can take the place of meat, fish, or fowl.)
2. Milk and milk products; Children—3 cups
                                         Teen-agers—4 cups
                                           Adults—2 cups
   Milk, cheese, and other milk-made foods, fortified soy milk.
3. Vegetables and fruits; four or more servings. A citrus or other vitamin C-rich fruit, highly colored green, red, or yellow vegetables.
4. Breads and cereals; four or more servings.
   Whole grain or enriched.

Simple food selected from these four basic groups and eaten in adequate amounts on a daily basis will provide you with excellent nourishment. There will be no need to buy highly advertised food supplements. Real food tastes better, too!

A variety of fresh fruit should play an important role in any carefully planned diet. It is considered a "protective" food, because it supplies nutrients to help ward off disease and to maintain optimum health. Since fruit is easy to digest, it is especially good for the evening meal, which should be light and easy for the stomach to handle. You may be interested to know that Americans consume more bananas than any other single fruit, on the average a little more than eighteen pounds per person per year. Maybe it's that zipper skin.

Don't feed your drain

A properly balanced diet will also include a variety of vegetables. Whenever possible these should be fresh, and prepared largely free from grease. Don't let the faddists convince you that all of them have to be eaten raw, even though this is a good way to use many of them. Actually, some vegetables are more easily digested when they are cooked. The main thing is not to *overcook* them. Use a minimum of water, and don't toss the remaining broth down the drain. You need the vitamins and minerals it contains a lot more than does your garbage disposal.

Natural is best

As much as possible, it is best to use foods in their natural state. Because of the great demand for convenience foods that "keep well," more than half of the total calories in the American diet are derived from highly refined foods. That adds up to poor nutrition. Let's take note, for instance, of what we have done to our breakfast cereals.

Bread with that something extra

Aboard ship in the South Pacific during World War II, we were once served some very unusual white bread. Each slice contained a number of small, pink circles about the size of a dime. Upon closer inspection we discovered in the center of each circle the body of a weevil; the pink halo was the result of his having been baked alive. I don't know whether the baker was unable to find a sieve, or whether he just didn't care. Most likely the latter. We must have been battle toughened as most everyone ate the bread, and that without much comment. Today, woe be to the weevil who saunters across my wife's kitchen counter.

In some ways, weevils are a lot smarter than people. They always turn up their nose at a canister of white flour as long as there is whole-wheat flour available. Weevils know where real nutrition is to be found.

Unfortunately, the best part of a kernel of wheat spoils first, the germ and the bran. In order to produce flour that keeps easily, we remove this most valuable portion and settle for the remainder, which is mostly starch. In the process we lose 77 per cent of the vitamin B_1, 60 per cent of the calcium, 70 per cent of the phosphorus, and 75 per cent of the iron. And where does all this lost goodness end up? We feed it to our cows and pigs so they can grow up to be stronger and healthier than our children! Who says truth isn't stranger than fiction.

This same loss occurs when we degerminate corn meal or any other cereal. As a boy visiting the farm, I remember that the rats in the corn crib were very selective. As long as there was plenty to eat they merely chewed the heart (germ) out of each kernel. As human beings we do just the opposite. Could rats and pigs be smarter than humans?

But what about enriched white bread? Doesn't the enrichment process put back what has been lost in the milling? Dr. Mervyn G. Hardinge of Loma Linda University warns:

"Unfortunately, our knowledge is not yet sufficient to know what is contained in the portion that is milled away. Of the twenty or more nutrients that are removed, enrichment is required to put back only three vitamins and iron." [5]

When you select your bread from the grocer's shelf, be sure to pick a loaf that is "100 per cent whole wheat." If the wrapper merely says "whole wheat," you may be buying enriched white bread with a pinch of whole-wheat flour and some dark food coloring. Wheat-germ bread is another good product.

Better yet, why not join the increasing number of people who are baking their own homemade wheat bread? Some invest in equipment that will even do the kneading for you. Be forewarned, however. Once your family catches the aroma of those beautiful golden loaves just out of the oven, you'll never again be able to satisfy them with the pallid, puffed-up substitute.

Want to see for yourself? Here's a simple recipe that will turn even the man of the house into a master baker. If your first effort is not so successful, remember practice makes perfect.

Basic Whole-Wheat Bread*

    1 package dry yeast (1 cake compressed; 1 tbsp. in bulk)
2-1/2 cups lukewarm water
    3 tbsp. honey
    1 cup enriched white flour
2-1/2 tsp. salt
    3 tbsp. oil
    5 to 6 cups whole-wheat flour (use only amount
        needed)

1. Add yeast to 1/2 cup of warm water.
2. In large bowl dissolve the honey in 2 cups warm water.
3. Add the softened yeast, white flour, and 1-1/2 cups whole-wheat flour. Stir till smooth.
4. Let this sponge rise until it is bubbly. Then add the remaining ingredients, stirring to a medium-stiff dough.
5. Turn out on a floured board and knead until the dough is smooth and elastic—6 to 10 minutes. Add flour as needed.
6. Place the dough in a warm, slightly oiled bowl; turn oiled side up and cover with damp cloth.
7. Set to rise in a warm place, and let rise until double in bulk.
8. Knead down and let rise again or shape into loaves and put immediately into the pans.
9. Let rise until nearly double in bulk. (A simple test is to press the dough lightly with the finger. If a slight depression remains, it is ready for the oven.)
10. Preheat oven to 400° F. Bake bread at this temperature for the first 10 minutes. Lower heat to 350° F. and finish baking at least 45 to 50 minutes more.

Yield: 2 loaves

---

* For white bread, substitute 5 to 6 cups enriched white flour for the whole-wheat flour.

Who knows, if the good word gets around, bread may once again become the staff of life.

Ever milk a bean?

Many people find their bodies do not tolerate milk, and with infants particularly this can be a serious problem. Modern food scientists have come to the rescue with a palatable milk made from soy beans. In its fortified form it is just as healthful as what Bossy provides down at the dairy. And since it is not an animal product, the human system does not react adversely to it.

It is encouraging that more and more mothers are breast-feeding their infants. Cow's milk is a good food, but it was designed especially for baby cows. For most infants nothing is as good as breast-feeding. It provides the correct dosage of all nutrients at low cost, protects the vulnerable infant with anti-infective agents, and ensures emotional support at the time when mental development is at its most rapid and critical stage. The relationship does things for the mother also.

The fat of the land

Fats add to the pleasure of eating and are essential for the absorption of such fat-soluble vitamins as A, D, K, and E. They are, however, the most concentrated source of energy in our diet, and thus should be used only in moderation. No more than 20 to 25 per cent of our daily calories should be in the form of fats.

And we should be aware of what *kind* of fats we are eating. A high level of cholesterol (a white, fatty crystalline alcohol) in the blood stream is one of several risk factors in heart disease. The amount of cholesterol in the blood is *decreased* by eating vegetable oils (polyunsaturated fatty acids) and *increased* by the use of saturated fatty acids found in meat, dairy products, and eggs. (Coconut oil is an exception; it also is saturated.) For all cooking, use vegetable oils that are liquid at room temperature. If such oils are hydrogenated, or hardened, they are not as beneficial.

Instead of drinking whole milk, it's a good idea to use low-fat or even skim milk. Budget-conscious consumers should be aware that non-fat powdered milk is perhaps the very best food bargain available.

And forget the butter; instead use one of the soft margarines on the market. These contain unsaturated fats, and thus are more desirable.

Sugar and spice, not so nice . . .

Condiments such as mustard, pepper, strong spices, vinegar, pickles, and chowchow are best left alone. They inflame the delicate lining of the stomach and make the blood feverish and impure. A little seems to call for more, until so many condiments are used that the food itself can scarcely be tasted. As the human system is thus irritated, a craving is created for something stronger and still stronger.

In order to be fit, our bodies demand a certain amount of salt, but most people use too much. The average American consumes 12-15 grams of salt daily, about three times as much as he needs.[6] To salt one's food before tasting it is a bad habit. Shaking the salt container too vigorously can result in health problems, not the least of which is high blood pressure.

Recently housewives were complaining about the high price of sugar, but in the thirteenth and fourteenth centuries a working man had to part with an entire week's wages for a single pound of the sweet stuff. For health's sake, it's too bad the price ever came down.

We've already mentioned the harmful effect excess sugar has upon dental health. Research also indicates a high sugar intake significantly increases blood cholesterol, and this in turn may be implicated in the incidence of heart disease.

Since the brain depends exclusively on glucose (a simple sugar) for its metabolism, anything that upsets the sugar content of the blood stream affects the operation of the brain cells. I know a young boy who was having such severe mental problems that his parents took him to a psychiatric hospital for testing. It turned out that the problem was an imbalance of sugar in his blood; as soon as this was corrected, through diet, his behavioral problem was solved.

Invitation to trouble

Whether you are aware of it or not, some of your best friends are white blood cells. Whenever germs invade your body, an army of these shock troops rushes to the scene and literally begins to eat the germs alive. These defense soldiers are tough. It is estimated that a single white blood cell can destroy about 14 enemy bacteria.

Great, as long as the defenders can do their thing properly. But just indulge in six teaspoonfuls of sugar and a white blood cell can handle only ten bacteria. Eleven teaspoonfuls and he can only cope with five. Eighteen teaspoonfuls and your white blood cell is weakened until he can just barely finish off two bacteria. Raise your sugar intake to twenty-four teaspoonfuls and he's down to one—real hand-to-hand combat.

Now you can see why some people are ill much of the time. Those who eat a lot of sugar are wide open to many of the infectious diseases that are going around.

Maybe you feel that because you don't heap those white crystals on top of everything in sight you don't use much sugar. The trouble is that much of the sugar we indulge in is well hidden. Do you know there are eleven teaspoonfuls lurking in a bottle of grape soda? Ten in a slice of iced chocolate cake, eight in a piece of apple pie, and even a half teaspoonful in a stick of chewing gum?

And don't let Junior choose his own cereals at the supermarket. Remember, he has been brainwashed from watching the ads that accompany kiddie programs on television. One popular dry cereal that claims to be loaded with vitamins and natural goodness is actually *more than 50 per cent sugar!*

Anything that tastes sweet contains sugar unless it is artificially sweetened with saccharin or cyclamate—and, if you've been reading, you know these last two items are also under suspicion. For truly natural sweetness why not put the sugar bowl away permanently and depend on raisins, dates, figs, and various fruits? It's not necessary to ban all sugar. In our home we use only a modest amount, and then only on weekends.

Don't be fooled into thinking the problem is solved merely by switching over to honey, raw sugar, or brown sugar. Although these substances may contain a few more minerals, the difference is not really significant as far as nutrition is concerned. Sugar is simply too unbalanced a food; too high in calories for the good it can do. Other foods provide an abundance of minerals and vitamins without an excess of calories from sucrose alone.

So the next time you are tempted to reach for a glazed doughnut, in the interest of good health reach instead for a juicy red apple or some other natural dessert from nature's storehouse.

1 Nathan J. Smith, M.D., "Americans: Foods and Foibles," *Life and Health*, March, 1974, p. 14.

2 Allan R. Magie, Ph.D., "Organic Foods," *Life and Health*, February, 1973, p. 25.

3 C. G. King, "Latest Advances in Nutrition," *Journal of the American Dietetic Association* 38: 223, 1961.

4 News Release (Chicago, Illinois: American Dietetic Association), March, 1975, p. 2.

5 Mervyn G. Hardinge, M.D., "Weevils Are Smarter Than People," *Life and Health*, August, 1972, p. 6.

6 William B. Kannel, M.D., "The Disease of Living," *Nutrition Today*, May/June, 1971, p. 10.

14

THE SICK CHICKEN
GOES FIRST

ANYONE WHO really wants to go all out in seeking good health and long life ought to seriously consider the possibility of becoming a vegetarian. Although such an approach to diet is ancient, today vegetarianism is enjoying a new wave of popularity. Many are beginning to see the wisdom of obtaining their nutrition firsthand from plant life rather than secondhand through the flesh of animals.

Perhaps I should explain what I mean by the term "secondhand." Only plants have the unique ability to manufacture food from the elements with the use of the sun's energy. No animal can do this. Experience has proved it is not only less expensive but also healthier to go right to the source of all this goodness, the plant itself.

"But surely you can't expect a laboring man to turn out a hard day's work on nothing but bread, beans, and apples!" Why not? In the animal kingdom the real beasts of burden are those that eat only plants. The big killer cat is great on short bursts of energy, but it is the ox, the horse, the camel that have staying power. If the elephant not only survives but performs astounding feats of strength while eating nothing but foliage, it stands to reason that a man might be able to do well on fruits and vegetables. Dr. Frederick J. Stare, professor of nutrition at Harvard University and world authority on diet, has stated plainly, "Lumberjacks may demand plenty of red meat, but that demand rests on habit and not on nutritional or medical basis."

The acid test

The real test of strength is endurance; how long can one's muscles do their task before giving up in exhaustion? The first experiment of this kind was carried on in the early part of this century. Vegetarian and nonvegetarian students were tested to see how many times they could squeeze a grip meter with their right hand. The vegetarians won handily with an average of 69 over the nonvegetarians average of 38. In a similar experiment even the *maximum* record of the nonvegetarians was barely more than *half* that of the vegetarians.[1]

More recently a Swedish scientist tested nine trained athletes on a stationary bicycle apparatus. Their assignment was to pump the pedals until their leg muscles were no longer able to respond. After three days on a high fat and protein diet (meat, eggs, fish, cheese, et cetera) the men ran out of steam after 57 minutes.

Next these very same athletes were tested following three days on a mixed diet such as eaten by the average person. This time they nearly doubled their previous record for an average of 114 minutes.

These same men went on a strictly vegetarian diet (high in carbohydrates), and this time they were able to hold out for 167 minutes—nearly three times as long as on the largely meat diet! No wonder some of the world's greatest athletes have been vegetarians. Why should *you* settle for second best?

But what about protein?

This is usually the first question raised in connection with a vegetarian regimen, and since protein is so vital to our well-being it deserves a clear-cut answer.

Back in the 1800's a Professor Karl von Voit of the University of Munich studied the food intake of 1,000 German laborers and determined their average protein consumption was 118 grams per day. He then hypothesized, incorrectly, that if workingmen were taking in this much protein daily, that must represent their actual *need*. This finding was accepted as the standard for protein intake for many, many years, but now we know better. Today the recommended protein allowance is only 56 grams for a man and 46 for a woman. Even that small amount is known to be twice or more the minimum requirement.[2]

Dr. Hardinge of Loma Linda University, and Harvard's Dr. Stare, did the most complete studies of people using different kinds of vegetarian diets. They found that both total vegetarians (those using no animal products) and lacto-ovo-vegetarians (those using milk and eggs) were actually eating *more* protein than was recommended by the Food and Nutrition Board of the National Research Council in Washington, D.C.[3] Dr. Hegsted of Harvard adds, "It is most unlikely that protein deficiency will develop in healthy adults on a diet in which cereals and vegetables supply adequate calories."[4]

Protein quality

"So much for the *amount* of protein, but what about quality?" Here again recent research indicates former fears were not well grounded:

"Formerly, vegetable proteins were classified as second-class and regarded as inferior to first-class proteins of animal origin; but this distinction has now been generally discarded. Certainly some vegetable proteins, if fed as the *sole* source of protein, are of relatively low value for promoting growth; but many field trials have shown that the proteins provided by suitable mixtures of vegetable origin enable children to grow as well as children provided with milk and other animal products.[5]

Bressani and Behar have stated:

"From a nutritional point of view, animal or vegetable proteins should not be differentiated. It is known today that the relative concentration of the amino acids, particularly of the essential ones, is the most important factor determining the biological value of a protein. . . . By combining different proteins in appropriate ways, vegetable proteins cannot be distinguished nutritionally from those of animal origin." [6]

Another possible problem comes to mind, however. Although a vegetarian who also uses milk has no trouble obtaining an adequate supply of vitamin B_{12}, we do not presently know of any practical source of this vitamin in plant food alone. Some individuals appear to maintain good health on a total vegetarian diet, while others experience some difficulty. Until further research makes things clear, the pure vegetarian should use fortified soybean milk or a vitamin B_{12} supplement.

Not only has it been shown that a vegetarian diet is on a par with a flesh diet but in many respects it is superior. There are some real risks connected with a flesh diet.

Animal fats have something that vegetable fats do not have—cholesterol. We have already mentioned the fact that cholesterol is linked with America's number one killer, coronary heart disease.

Another somewhat unpleasant thought is that at any given time animals have in their flesh, waste products on the way to the kidneys. Anyone eating this flesh is merely adding the animal's waste products to his own, thus putting an extra work load on his own kidneys.

Still another disadvantage is fatigue, a common complaint. Remember those nine Swedish athletes who could pedal only a third as long on a meat diet as they could on a nonflesh diet.

Marketing disease

Perhaps the most serious consideration is that the animal kingdom has become one vast reservoir of diseases, many of which can be passed along to man. James Steele has pointed out, "Of more than 200 communicable diseases of animals, one-half are considered infectious to man, and more than 80 are transmitted naturally between vertebrate animals and man." [7]

I was raised in the Midwest where much of our poultry and livestock are raised, and I know from personal experience that it is the sick bird or critter that goes to market first. When that hen has a badly drooping wing, or that cow has an advanced case of "cancer eye," it is time to move fast. Buyers won't purchase dead animals—but they will take them if they're still breathing. A rancher once showed me some white spots in the eye of a cow, stating it was the beginning of cancer eye. He indicated this particular animal would be sent off with his very next shipment. Later I asked a veterinarian what he did for a critter with an advanced state of cancer eye. He nonchalantly explained, "First I take a ladle and scoop out the entire eye and orbit. Then I pack the cavity full of sulfa [this was some years ago], sew the eyelid shut, and advise the rancher to get the animal to market fast."

"But isn't meat inspected so we can know it is safe?" This question is well answered by *Life and Health's* special supplement Vegetarianism:

"There are not enough veterinarians to do the inspecting, so lay people are utilized—with very meager training. Often these lay inspectors are asked to examine each day as many as one thousand or more fowl and a hundred or more cattle!

"How many human bodies could a pathologist examine in one day? Probably not more than three or four and then never without a microscopic examination. Obviously those who examine animals are supposed to do the impossible. They are expected to study large animals without even the benefit of a microscope.

"And when cancer is found in the animals, what is done? It is removed; but what about the rest of the carcass? It is usually passed for food. Those who know something about the spread of cancers realize that the removal of a tumor does not necessarily remove all cancerous cells. The blood or lymphatic system already may have spread such cells to other parts of the body." [8]

I should point out that it has not yet been proved that animals can transmit cancer to man, although scientists expect momentarily to find such proof. It would seem only a matter of time. Anyway, we already know, beyond the shadow of a doubt, of many other diseases that are transmitted.

Let me mention another bit of discomforting news. It was recently determined that in a little more than two pounds of charcoal broiled steak there's as much *benzo(a)pyrene* as in the smoke from 600 cigarettes![9] So? Benzo(a)pyrene is a cancer-stimulating agent; when fed to mice they develop stomach tumors and leukemia.

"But maybe these substances develop cancer only in mice, not humans?" Maybe. But researchers suspect otherwise, and I personally would rather not run the risk. The reason these strongly held suppositions are difficult to prove is that we cannot experimentally inject into human beings substances we believe cause cancer.

There is also the problem of keeping meat once it is processed. About half the beef sold in the United States is in the form of hamburger. The Consumers Union tested 250 hamburger samples from various retailers for bacteria—coliform—whose presence usually indicates fecal contamination. And such contamination in turn may mean the meat contains disease-causing organisms. Consumers Union judged that 73 per cent of the samples had a coliform count high enough to be the possible cause of mild illness. They also determined that 20 per cent of the 126 ready-ground samples had a total-bacteria count high enough to qualify them as already beginning to spoil.[10]

The vegetarian is happy to sit down to his meal and not have to wonder what it died from.

Flesh foods and world hunger

Those of us living in a land of plenty are just now beginning to realize that Spaceship Earth has its limitations. Unless we all begin to face up to the hard facts of supply and demand, unprecedented famines will be a reality in the near future.

One practical approach to the problem is to lower the demand for food, to cease bringing into the world more lives than our earth can properly support. Another solution is to increase the supply of available food. No doubt attention should be given to both possibilities.

Much has already been done to increase plant yield, but this, too, has its limitations. There is yet another factor to consider. Most of the world's millions already are, of necessity, virtual vegetarians. Meat is a luxury they can afford only occasionally. If all of us were vegetarians the food supply problem would be greatly eased.

As a food machine the cow (along with other food animals) is hopelessly inefficient. *For every 100 calories of plant food the cow consumes, it returns only one twenty-fifth—four lonely calories—in edible beef!*

Let's illustrate this inefficient use of plant life in yet another way. Here is a 12-year-old boy weighing 105 pounds. If he were to derive all of his energy from flesh food for a twelve-month period, it would require an equivalent of the meat from four calves. But do you know how much plant food it would take to fatten those four calves to a total weight of 2,250 pounds? Twenty million alfalfa plants, weighing 17,850 pounds! All for one small boy.[11]

In the populous Orient, people obtain their energy supply basically from vegetables. That means they are ten times more efficient in utilizing the earth's food supply than the people of the United States, who depend so much on animal products. More and more, concerned and thinking people are turning to a vegetarian way of life—and they are being rewarded by better health.

Don't panic, ladies

When a vegetable regimen is first proposed, the average housewife reacts with instant panic. Plenty of tender loving care is showered on the steak, but poorly prepared vegetables are often plopped on the plate merely to add color and take up space. Cooking vegetables attractively, healthfully, and deliciously is almost a lost art.

Of course, the utilization of some time and effort can bring the vegetables back into line, but what about that entree? The transition from flesh foods can be eased considerably by the use of *meat analogs*. These are all-vegetable products that look like, taste like, and have the consistency of meat. And we are not talking about some space-age idea still on the drawing board; these fascinating foods are already on the market. You may choose from a wide variety of foods that resemble chicken, turkey, beef, ham, sausage, bacon, skallops, wieners, hamburger, and others. Some of these products come in cans, while others are frozen.

In many cases these meat analogs are already to be found on your grocer's shelves. If not, you may contact one of the outlets listed on page 154.

As most housewives experienced in vegetarian cookery will attest, the very finest vegetarian entrees are those stirred up from scratch at home, using such items as beans, peas, or lentils in combination with cereal grains and vegetables. For recipe books featuring such delicious, taste-tested dishes turn to page 152.

I hope many readers will give serious consideration to becoming vegetarians, but it is not a step to be taken lightly. Although not really a difficult transition, such a decision should be based on solid knowledge. For a sensible, scientific, and highly attractive treatment of the subject, written especially for laymen, see page 151.

---

[1] I. Fisher, *Yale Medical Journal,* March, 1907.

[2] D. M. Hegsted, "Minimum Protein Requirements of Adults," *American Clinical Nutrition,* 1968, 21:352.

[3] Food and Nutrition Board—National Research Council, *Recommended Dietary Allowance,* 7th edition, National Academy of Sciences Publication 1964, Washington, D.C., 1968.

[4] D. M. Hegsted, A. G. Tsongas, D. B. Abbot, and F. J. Stare, "Protein Requirements of Adults," *J. Lab. Clin. Med.,* 1946, 31:261.

[5] "New Sources of Protein," *Lancet,* vol. 2, 1959, p. 956.

[6] R. Bressani and M. Behar, in E. S. Livingston (ed.), Proc. 6th Intl. Congress of Nutrition, 1964, p. 182.

[7] James H. Steele, "Infectious Diseases Common to Animals and Man," *Consumer Reports,* August, 1971, p. 14.

[8] *Life and Health* Supplement, *Vegetarianism,* 1973, pp. 16, 17.

[9] W. Lijinsky and P. Shubik, "Benzo(a)pyrene and other polynuclear hydrocarbons in charcoal-broiled meat." *Science,* 145:53, 55, 1964.

[10] "A Close Look at Hamburgers," *Consumer Reports,* August, 1971, p. 479.

[11] Allan R. Magie, Ph.D., and Almer A. Widmer, Ph.D., "The Real Energy Crisis Is a Cow," *Life and Health,* September, 1973, p. 20.

THE
BATTLE
OF THE BULGE

THE CUISINE aboard our gunboat during World War II left a lot to be desired. The "cook" was usually conscripted from among those crew members who lacked either the mentality or ambition to learn any of the other specialties aboard. Not surprisingly, these unwilling chefs were not noted for putting their entire heart into their work.

In all fairness, I should say they didn't have much to work with. The galley was designed to prepare food for a crew of twenty, but eventually had to serve sixty-five. It was hardly larger than an oversized telephone booth, and in high seas a cook was lucky to come through uninjured, let alone turn out works of art.

Because our assignments kept us far from the supply centers, we almost never saw anything fresh. Dehydrated foods were in the experimental stage; powdered milk stayed gritty even after mixing, mashed potatoes looked (and tasted) like wallpaper paste. Even a blowtorch couldn't phase the waxy margarine concocted especially for hot climates. We survived largely on ship-baked whole-wheat bread and peanut butter— fortunately a nutritious combination.

I believe we were reasonably healthy, but our daily calorie intake was very low. Always pencil-thin before the war, I came out of the conflict looking like Mohandas Gandhi just after one of his longer fasts. Then came the reintroduction to home cooking, and the result was I shot up to 199 pounds almost overnight. This didn't bother me too much until I learned someone had referred to me as "the fat man with the mustache." That really shook me up. Something had to go, and I decided it should be the extra weight I had put on.

Today we have an avalanche of information on good nutrition. Even back then my wife had received sensible advice somewhere. She put me on a calorie count. That is, she calculated a daily calorie quota that would cause me to lose weight slowly, but surely. No kooky diet ideas were involved. I ate pretty much the foods I was used to, except that portions were carefully controlled. When my plate was empty I left the table; there were never any seconds. If there were a few lonesome little calories I hadn't used, the amount was written on a slip of paper and placed in a cup. When the calories in the cup added up to a treat, I could enjoy one without having it affect my weight reduction program. The plan worked beautifully; my weight came down and stayed down.

Mirror, mirror on the wall

Sometimes it seems as though most of the people in the United States are either just starting on a weight reduction program, are in the middle of one, or have just given up on one. Approximately 30 per cent of our adult population is overweight, and obesity is a real malnutrition problem in this land of plenty. The number of those who could be considered obese has doubled since 1950!

Are you wondering just where you fit into the picture? Science now has some sophisticated ways of differentiating between muscle and fat, but Dr. Jean Mayer suggests a common sense method: "The easiest and most obvious way is to look at yourself naked in a mirror. If you *look* fat you probably *are* fat." [1]

Now suppose the mirror tells us plainly it is time to shed a few unneeded and unwanted pounds. Where to begin? First of all, forget the usual excuses such as the one about "problem glands." There is a gland problem in obese persons; it involves, frankly, the overworked salivary glands. Excuses may ease feelings of guilt, but they don't change the reading on the scales.

Resist the temptation to take off on one of those crash diets we listed previously. You probably added those extra pounds slowly over a long period of time; it may take a while to lose them safely. A pound a week is fast enough. If you are grossly obese and feel the need for something more drastic, work out a special program with your doctor. Don't attempt it on a "do it yourself" basis.

Also avoid seeking a miracle in a bottle of pills. Or any combination of pills. This route is thought to have caused the death of six women in a single State. The "easy" way may be the hardest way of all.

To really simplify the problem, think of it in terms of a banking transaction. If you deposit more money than you draw out, your account is bound to grow—and, of course, the exact opposite is true, as well. Similarly, if you take in more food calories than you expend in your daily activity, those extra calories are going to be stored as fat—usually in the wrong places.

Now, if you are an active person and do not take in enough food calories to maintain that activity, your body will be forced to draw energy from the fat you have stored. In other words, you lose weight. The ideal is to get your weight into the proper range, and then keep your account in balance.

Now if we have been a bit careless and have too much in the "calorie bank," how do we begin a sensible reducing program? Here are a few helpful suggestions:

First of all, plan to cut down on your total calorie intake. Since they are going to be limited, each calorie becomes rather precious and should represent good nutrition. That means sugar is to be virtually eliminated from the diet; the calories in sugar are simply too expensive, nutritionally speaking.

Second, cut down on the total intake of fats, and especially try to avoid animal fats. Go easy on any fats that are solid at room temperature.

Next, slow up on the snack foods; the fewer the better. Pretzels, soft drinks, and potato chips represent "empty" calories. You can't afford them.

Cut back on the size of the portions on your plate. No matter how carefully selected and nutritious the food, too *much* of it spells trouble.

The mode of food preparation is important too. A simple baked potato boasts only a hundred calories, but mashing it with added milk may push it to 150 calories. Now if you like plenty of butter on your potatoes, think in terms of 250 calories. You can even better that mark with French fries. If you are trying for a record, then hashbrowns made with animal fat could push it up into the 400-calories-plus zone. And potato chips may peak at a frightening 800! See what we mean? If you are really serious about keeping your weight in line, it might be a good idea to settle for the simple baked potato with maybe a dash of margarine.

Determine to eat absolutely nothing between meals. Literally tons of our nations's unwanted poundage is added as a result of nibbling before the TV set.

Try not to serve too great a variety of foods at a single meal. To do so is to invite everyone to overeat.

You knew we were going to mention desserts, didn't you? More expensive calories. Try to avoid the lure of cakes, pies, ice cream, and cookies. Instead, enjoy a piece of naturally sweet fresh fruit. An added bonus is that the latter will serve as a dental detergent, a very pleasant way of brushing your teeth.

Eat a good breakfast

If you are interested in reducing, never try to accomplish it by skipping breakfast. If any meal of the day is to be omitted let it be the evening meal. You need food in the morning to supply energy for the day. And those early morning calories are more apt to be burned up than the ones you indulge in late at night. The latter are more apt to show up as unwanted fat.

And be sure you have a *good* breakfast. Real whole-grain cereal. Low-fat or skim milk. A handful of raisins or dates stirred in rather than sugar. Whole-wheat toast. Peanut butter, or a handful of nuts. Orange juice. Some additional fruit. With a start like that, you may have trouble keeping your feet on the ground.

The danger of baby fat

Chubby babies may be cute, but U.S. Public Health Service studies show obese boys and girls tend to grow up to be fat adults, less able than others to lose fat or to maintain fat loss. Those who become obese before 10 years of age often seem destined to remain that way. If your youngsters have an overweight problem help them to slim down *now* while it is much easier.

This is vital

Here's a simple formula you might keep in mind:

Excess calories + lack of exercise = overweight.

We have talked of the need to cut back on extra calories, but equally important in the life of the average American is the need for more physical activity. Attacking the weight problem from both directions will prove most rewarding. Actually, even though you are a bit overweight, you may not be eating too much right now. It may be that you are merely eating too much for your degree of *activity*. Dr. U. D. Register of Loma Linda University warns:

"To gain weight we must eat more than we use; *to lose weight, we must use more than we eat.* And it is most difficult to eat less than we use unless we get enough exercise. In fact, a person who tries to lose weight by diet alone is almost certainly doomed to be hungry the rest of his life." [2]

Not a very pleasant prospect. On the other hand, Dr. George Mann, of Vanderbilt University, promises:

"Be fit and active and you can pretty well eat what you wish." [3]

You may be wondering, "What kind of 'activity' should I

engage in to help keep my weight down?" Perhaps the best exercise for this particular purpose would be a *brisk* walk of at least 30 minutes, four or five days a week. This exercises the large muscle groups and raises the heart rate a reasonable amount. Such an effort should leave one a bit out of breath and should also cause one to perspire.

I have met people, and so have you, who can put away an astonishing amount of food without gaining weight. This doesn't mean, however, that they are escaping unscathed. Overeating is a bad habit any way you look at it. Even though one may not become obese, the stomach is often exhausted, and the digestive organs enfeebled. Precious vital force is depleted, and mental dullness is the order of the day. In eating, as with other things, moderation is the key to good health.

If you would like to read more about solving the problem of overweight or obesity, note the easy-to-read study offered on page 151.

A closing thought: You're not interested in a yo-yo experience; a lifelong battle with the bathroom scale. What you are looking for is a permanent answer to the problem. Loma Linda University's Dr. John Scharffenberg has some words of wisdom that should be heeded:

"*Don't go on a diet!* If you think you're on a diet, you'll just be waiting for the day when you can get off that diet and go back to eating. What you need is a right way of eating, a permanent way of life." [4]

Good advice indeed. A new and better way of eating and drinking for today and every day from now on.

---

[1] J. Mayer, Ph.D., *Overweight: Causes, Cost, and Control* (Inglewood Cliffs, New Jersey: Prentice Hall, 1968).

[2] U. D. Register, Ph.D., "Keeping Your Calorie 'Bank' in Balance," *Life and Health* Supplement, *Obesity,* 1974, p. 47.

[3] George V. Mann, M.D., "Obesity—The Other Side of the Coin," *Ibid.,* p. 18.

[4] John Scharffenberg, M.D., "I'm Obese—What Can I Do?" *Ibid.,* p. 32.

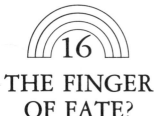

THE FINGER
OF FATE?

"I'M A LITTLE nervous. My surgery is scheduled for tomorrow morning." The patient, propped up against two thick
pillows, wheezed as he spoke. Every other sentence was punc-
tuated by a series of racking coughs that threatened to tear
apart his already emaciated form. As chaplain of a large hospital in Karachi, Pakistan, I offered my sympathy along with
a bit of encouragement. Staring at me quietly for a moment,
he shrugged and gave a one-word reply, "Kismet," the word in
his language for fate.

This gentleman's analysis of his predicament certainly is
not unique to his part of the world. Over here we refer to our
"luck," either good or bad. If we win a free basket of groceries
it's good luck; if we end up in the hospital with an illness it's
bad luck. Our own Western brand of kismet.

But at least as far as illness is concerned, I want to fly in
the face of this it's-not-my-fault-and-why-did-it-have-to-hap-
pen-to-me psychology. The blunt truth is that the great ma-
jority of patients in our hospitals have put themselves there,
either deliberately or through ignorance. There is no real mystery about the problem at all.

Disease never comes without a cause. The way is prepared, and disease is actually invited, by a disregard of the

laws of health. Nature bears a surprising amount of abuse without apparent resistance, but finally arouses herself and makes a determined effort to remove the effects of the ill-treatment she has suffered. Her effort to correct these conditions often manifests itself in fever or some other form of sickness.

A concise definition of disease might then be: "Disease is an effort of nature to free the system from conditions that result from a violation of the laws of health."

There, I did it; I used what many today seem to consider a bad word "laws." The emphasis is rather on unfettered freedom, "doing one's own thing" without interference. It hasn't worked out too well. In fact, many are beginning to realize there is no true freedom without law; only chaos. Cast several strangers onto a deserted island, and within a few days they will of necessity have set up a system of rules and regulations.

But right now we are more concerned with the laws of nature than the laws of men. Whether we like them or not, or whether we even believe in them at all, these natural laws exist. Take for instance the law of gravity, which is manifested by the tendency of material bodies to fall toward the center of the earth. Some place in this old world there may be a man who simply doesn't believe in the law of gravity. Nevertheless, if he throws a ball straight up into the air he had better duck because it is going to come right back down again. Or suppose that he, with courage of his convictions, confidently steps off the balcony of an eighty-story building. His impact with the street will prove just as fatal as that of one who *does* believe in the law of gravity. That law is continually in operation, influenced not one bit by the opinions of mere men.

So it is with the laws of health. They are written on every nerve and sinew of man, and we disregard them only at our peril. To break these laws is to invite the sure result: sickness.

In times past we transgressed in ignorance because our knowledge of how the human system worked was limited. We still had much to learn about germs and infection. Nothing at all was known about viruses. As a boy, I still remember the red quarantine sign on the front of our home warning one and all to beware of the measles. An even more dreaded sign was the one announcing smallpox. How much medical science has learned since those days!

But that is not to say we have moved into a Utopian era of good health. Our hospitals are as crowded as ever, and we still suffer the usual quota of aches and pains. Anyone living to a hundred still rates a special write-up. Although we have brought many of our infectious diseases under control, we still fall before the degenerative ones. And where we once could plead ignorance, we now know very well what is killing us. It is our life-style, our deliberate disregard of the laws of health. Let's take note of several common habits that demonstrate the typical pattern of *cause and effect:*

Alcohol

Sunday morning in lower Manhattan's Bowery is like Sunday morning nowhere else. One simply has to see it to believe it. I had read descriptions of "skid row," so I anticipated the bleary-eyed, stubble-chinned derelicts stumbling along the street. But the numbers overwhelmed me. Inert, vomit-stained bodies were strewn everywhere; across the sidewalk, propped up in doorways, and in the gutters. Scores and scores of them, block after block. It was one of the most dismal and depressing scenes I have ever witnessed. The bottom of America's barrel.

Well, not quite. There is one more step down. Some years ago I managed to wangle a visit to the famed Bellevue morgue. Again I wasn't quite prepared for the overwhelming body count involved. Row after row of lockers stretched from floor to high ceiling. And each one, as my guide graphically proved by opening a door and pulling out a metal deck, contained a refrigerated corpse. At one end of the room was a traffic jam of wheeled stretchers. On top of each, covered with a length of butcher paper, was yet another body awaiting processing.

Business is especially brisk at the Bellevue morgue, because all unidentified bodies from New York's five boroughs are brought here. Many are eventually identified and removed by relatives; many others remain forever nothing more than a statistic on a government form. Free burial is provided in a potter's field on a nearby island.

I'm quite sure some of you are thinking: "Oh, come on. You know that what you have described in the Bowery represents only a very small portion of those who drink. And scare tactics have never been very successful. I'm strictly a social drinker, myself."

You're right. The bums on skid row represent no more than 5 per cent of all the citizens who indulge in beverage alcohol. And for some reason, scare tactics *don't* seem to be very effective in changing human behavior. The odds are that you'll never end up stumbling along the Bowery or Chicago's State Street, although it's a possibility.

About one in ten of the 95 million Americans who drink is now either a full-fledged alcoholic or at least a problem drinker.

Anyway, let's turn our attention to this matter of social drinking, also known as "the cup that cheers." We are immediately faced with a paradox. The flood of hard drugs in our country during recent years has brutally torn the fabric of our society. Drug addiction has proved to be one of the most devastating and difficult problems ever faced by government. And unnumbered parents have been utterly shaken to find that a son or daughter is involved.

Now the paradox. Pale and tense, Dad shakes his head in unbelief as local authorities break the bad news. "I just can't understand it. Ours is a decent home. We've given our kids all the things they really needed, even though it meant a sacrifice on our part. How in the world could they let us down by getting into drugs?"

All the time Dad stands there explaining how excellent the home environment has been, he has a highball in one hand. He would never think of buying his son a syringe to mainline heroin, or of dropping him off at a pot party. But when Junior gets into the liquor cabinet Dad isn't too exercised. That's something entirely different—he thinks.

Let's face it; alcohol is a drug and a potent one at that. No matter how exquisite the decanter, or how pleasant sounding the brand name, alcohol is poison as far as the human system is concerned. Nature does her best to save us from ourselves, even in our ignorance. The body fights to ward off any noxious substance. That first smell of the real stuff (let's forget for the moment all the limes, lemons, oranges, tomato juice, olives, and myriad other legitimate foods used to make alcohol enjoyable or at least bearable) is enough to make many a novice gag. And that first swallow burns all the way down saying clearly, "Hold up. Something's wrong here." Even the stomach frequently gets in the act by rejecting the draft and sending it back up. A person has to work at taking on the drinking habit.

Of course, the body is a marvel at adjustment. Even something as deadly as strychnine can be reasonably well tolerated eventually if taken in tiny, ever-increasing dosages. The body will finally quit crying "Help," but that doesn't mean it isn't being damaged or even destroyed. There is still a day of reckoning.

Back to poor, confused Dad. Let's hope he is beginning to realize he himself laid the groundwork for the use of hard drugs in his family when he put his stamp of approval on a "softer" drug, namely alcohol. No wonder the kids consider liquor just one step up from soda pop and are turning to it in ever increasing numbers. Many of them have caught on that the hard drug scene is nowhere, oblivion. But plain alcohol, well that's an entirely different matter.

The most devastating drug

Dr. Morris Chafetz, director of the National Institute on Alcohol Abuse and Alcoholism, sees it in an entirely different light. He says, "Young people are moving from a wide range of other drugs to *the most devastating drug*—the one most widely misused of all—alcohol." Let's not be comforted because the youngsters are turning from cocaine to cocktails or from "bennies" to beer. The end result may be even worse.

Unfortunately, Mom may have "come a long way," too. Years ago the saloon with its sawdust covered floor was strictly a man's world. Now many women feel sufficiently liberated to join their male counterparts at the bar or cocktail lounge. In yet another area they are rapidly achieving equality; some parts of the country have a nearly identical ratio between male and female alcoholics.

The physical effects of beverage alcohol upon the human system are devastating. Alcohol degenerates and destroys liver cells, and may eventually bring on cirrhosis and death. Excessive use of alcohol is now being causatively linked with certain kinds of heart disease, and possibly with impotence. Because alcohol supplies ample calories but no food value, heavy drinkers are often malnourished.

Just as insidious as what alcohol does to man's physical well-being is how it affects his mental processes. Drinking is often used as a crutch for individuals who have problems adjusting socially. Alcohol passes from the stomach into the blood stream and from there into the central nervous system. The very first part of the brain to be affected is that part that controls personality and character. Inhibitions are lowered and a person's moral standards may suffer. A normally dignified individual may become argumentative and belligerent, or unbearably silly.

Now comes the frightening part. The motor centers of the brain eventually are affected; the person's reflexes become dulled and his ability to coordinate his movements impaired. But he *feels* confident and capable of handling most anything. If in this condition he climbs behind the wheel of an automobile he immediately becomes a potential murderer.

Some years ago I attended a service club meeting where the speakers for the day made a profound impression on all in attendance. It was good they were "after dinner" speakers. The two gentlemen presenting the program had been recipients of a government grant, their task being to study all highway fatalities within a certain part of the State over a period of three years. Even the police were not allowed to remove bodies from the wreckage until these men had arrived to make certain observations and record the scene on film.

The slides of the dead victims were in living color and we were all appalled at the carnage. After the program I approached one of the speakers and asked, "As a result of your studies, were you able to detect any common denominator in all these accidents?"

His reply was significant. "Only one. More than half of the victims had been drinking."

Citizens of the United States became understandably exercised about the tragic loss of life in the Vietnamese war. But we lose as many people in *one* year on our highways as we did in the entire *twelve* years of conflict in Vietnam! That grim war cost us more than 50,000 dead; our wreckage-strewn highways cost us 55,500 dead each year. Plus a million individuals who suffer major injuries. Let's keep in mind that "the cup that cheers" plays a vital role in this annual blood bath.

Not only does alcohol mix poorly with gasoline, but it doesn't do so well with water, either. Investigators from Johns Hopkins School of Public Health reported that in one metropolitan area 47 per cent of the drowning victims had been drinking alcohol.[1]

Recently it has been discovered that heavy liquor drinking can lead to a condition of hypoglycemia, or low blood sugar, with its numerous complications.[2] Alcoholic workers cost their employers from eight to ten billion dollars annually.[3] "After heart disease and cancer, alcoholism is the country's biggest health problem. On [the] average, an alcoholic's life span is shortened by 10 to 12 years."[4]

"In half of all murders in the United States, either the killer or the victim—or both—have been drinking."[5]

"A fourth of all suicides have significant amounts of alcohol in their bloodstreams."[6]

People who drink heavily are seven times more likely to be separated or divorced than the general population."[7]

With beverage alcohol leaving such a wide trail of death

and disease, why are we so reticent to speak out against it? Perhaps Carrie Nation and her hatchet-swinging cohorts gave the word *temperance* a bad aura. That's unfortunate, because temperance is basically a good word. The dictionary defines it as "the state or quality of being temperate; habitual moderation." I have an even better definition; one that all would do well to memorize:

"True temperance is total abstinence from that which is harmful, and a moderate use of that which is good."

There is only one truly safe course to follow as far as liquor is concerned, and that is to leave it strictly alone. Forget the social glass. Toast your friends with tomato juice. The reason some people are prone to become alcoholics is not yet fully known, but no one has ever become an alcoholic who refused to take that first drink.

For years we assumed that the brain damage suffered by alcoholics was simply one of the end effects of years of hard drinking. Recently we have learned that every time a person takes a few drinks he permanently damages his brain. A team of scientists headed by Dr. Melvin H. Knisely, professor of anatomy at the Medical University of South Carolina in Charleston, has discovered that drinking alcohol affects the red-blood cells. They become sticky and clump together forming a "sludge." As a result of this condition, life-giving oxygen cannot get through to the nerve cells. If deprived of oxygen for a mere three minutes these cells are seriously damaged; if this deprivation lasts for fifteen to twenty minutes they die.[8] Brain cells, unlike those of other parts of the body, are not replaced. Damage done to the brain, through the destruction of its cells, is irreversible.

Dr. Knisely admits to having been a moderate drinker, but no more. "There is only one way to be safe from the danger of alcohol," he declares. "That is to quit it cold."

The cost of liquor over the counter is high enough, but it is even more expensive in terms of its effect on health and well-being. A penalty is affixed to every violation of the laws of health, and sooner or later the bill must be paid.

Tobacco

My introduction to tobacco came, as is often the case, out behind the barn. The clandestine meeting involved two other young buddies, one of whom had come into possession of an entire carton of cigarettes. We had already tried sucking on a length of grapevine as well as cornsilk wrapped in brown paper, so felt we were ready for the real thing. We decided to go through the entire ten packs in one sitting, which turned out to be quite a challenge. Even though we soon settled for a mere two or three puffs on each cigarette, by the time we ground out the last butt each of us was thoroughly sick.

I don't know just what the giveaway was. It could have been nicotine-stained fingers, smoker's breath, a green complexion, or an obviously guilty conscience. Perhaps all four. At any rate, I soon experienced one of the unpleasant "side effects" of smoking; a belt vigorously applied to the backside. At the tender age of 10 I decided to give up the use of tobacco.

What happened behind that barn should have been an education in itself. My body was certainly attempting to tell me something as with watering eyes I hacked and coughed my way into a complete state of dizziness. My senses were trying to relay the message, "You must be confused. This stuff is poison!"

I don't think I have ever met a smoker who didn't get these warning messages. But most go charging right on past the caution lights, and the human body, in its wonderfully adaptive way, finally learns to tolerate the nicotine invasion. Eventually this toleration turns into a true addiction and another willing victim has been "hooked" on an exceedingly demanding habit.

Of course, things seem pleasant enough for a time. The poisons in tobacco are of the slow, insidious variety, and it may be fifteen or twenty years before serious consequences show up. By that time, unfortunately, many of the disease processes that have been developing cannot be reversed.

Smoking is an expensive habit, but the real cost is not calculated in dollars and cents. The actual cost must be figured in terms of the effects of the habit on the human mechanism. First of all, there is the matter of general fitness. All serious athletes realize that the man who doesn't indulge has a decided advantage over the one who does. Check out, for instance, the leading contenders in the annual foot race up Pike's Peak. You won't find a cigarette cough in a carload of them. Smokers who dare take on this demanding challenge are apt to be found sitting on a rock at timberline when the checkered flag comes down.

I don't know just how long you're planning on living, but if you are interested in staying around as long as possible don't get involved with the smoking habit. Or if you're already involved, get out. Cold, hard statistics indicate smokers die at a 68 per cent faster rate than nonsmokers. Or to break it down into even plainer language: every time a heavy smoker lights up, he is giving up six to nine minutes of his life span.

Hardening of the arteries

The greatest single killer in the United States today is arteriosclerosis, or hardening of the arteries. It accounts for more than half of all deaths caused by disease. The problem seems to be directly related to the American diet, which is high in fats. But recent studies show that substances in tobacco still further increase these fatty deposits inside the arteries, thus predisposing to heart trouble.

The problem is compounded because nicotine also causes spasm of the arteries, making it even more difficult for these vessels to carry life-giving blood to the various organs of the body. When hardening of the arteries narrows a blood vessel, potential disaster is close at hand. If the coronary artery is narrowed one may experience a heart attack; if an artery in the brain is narrowed the result may be a stroke. Not a very good choice in any case.

Although heart attacks were once considered almost exclusively a male problem, women seem determined to catch up. In a recent study involving women smokers who died suddenly from coronary heart disease, some rather sobering statistics came to light. Ten per cent of those who died were non-smokers, 28 per cent were light smokers, and 62 per cent were heavy smokers. The heavy smokers averaged a life span of only 48 years, while nonsmokers averaged 67 years—a significant advantage of 19 years.[9]

Emphysema

Speaking of ways to go, there is also emphysema, which now affects more than one-and-a-half million people in the United States. Substances in tobacco smoke irritate the delicate lining of the lungs until the walls of this organ's tiny air sacs burst and begin to form ever larger pockets. Finally there just isn't enough lung tissue surface left to efficiently make the all-important exchange of oxygen and carbon dioxide.

People afflicted with this particular disease are engaged in a constant battle to breathe. They have a continual sense of suffocation, and are too weak to be productive. Giving up the "weed" helps, of course, but the damage to lung tissue is irreversible. And the odds of facing this unpleasant prospect? In a careful study of men who died from various causes, some degree of "emphysema was present in 10 out of every 100 non-smokers, 53 out of every 100 pipe and cigar smokers, 87 out of every 100 light cigarette smokers, and more than 99 out of every 100 heavy cigarette smokers." [10]

Cancer

Perhaps one of the most feared words in the English language is "cancer." Here again tobacco plays a major role. Cancer of the throat, mouth, vocal cords, and esophagus are all more common among pipe, cigar, or cigarette smokers than among nonsmokers. Where tobacco really plays a starring role, however, is in connection with lung cancer—a form of the disease that is 95 per cent fatal. If you are a two-pack-a-day man, you are 15 to 20 times more apt to die of lung cancer than is your nonsmoking neighbor.

And even if you are one of the fortunate 5 per cent who survive lung cancer, it still isn't a cheerful picture. I person-

ally have stood in surgery to observe a lung removal at close
range. Just watching this major operation was traumatic
enough; I never want to be under the cutting edge of the
scalpel.

Hopefully, enough has been said already to discourage
merely switching from cigarettes to a pipe or cigars. The law
of cause and effect still operates, and although the odds may
be a bit better and the trouble sites may differ, the end results
are often the same.

Just a word on behalf of those too young to speak for
themselves. Mothers who smoke are more apt to have premature (by weight) babies or to lose them while they are still in
infancy. Children who have smoking fathers and mothers
have more frequent respiratory illnesses than those raised in
families where no one smokes.[11] Surely children ought to be
smoke free until they are old enough to decide for themselves
what they want to do with their lives.

You may have been thinking, "Well, this all sounds pretty
scary, but since I'm a nonsmoker myself none of it applies to
me." Wrong. Unless you live alone in a desert cave, I'm sure
you do some smoking whether you want to or not. When that
man in the seat next to you lights up you're involved. The
smoke he blows in your face isn't quite so bad because his lungs
have already filtered out part of the poison. However, the
smoke drifting directly your way from his idling cigarette contains even more carbon monoxide than the smoke he himself
is inhaling.

Increasingly it is being recognized that the nonsmoker has
a right to breathe uncontaminated air, and it is becoming easier
and easier to avoid smoking by proxy. If you are a nonsmoker,
in a courteous way it is time for you to stand up for your
rights.

Good news

Although most people who quit smoking do so on their
own, there is good news for those who feel the need of special
help. Thousands are kicking the habit each year through a

community program called the Five-Day Plan to Stop Smoking. This down-to-earth approach to the problem has proved highly successful in countries all around the world. It is frequently offered without charge as a community service. When a fee for material is requested it is only a minimal amount. To learn more about this plan and when a session will be available in your area, turn to page 152 in the Appendix.

It's all right there on the pack in plain English: "Warning: The Surgeon General Has Determined That Cigarette Smoking Is Dangerous to Your Health." A simple matter of cause and effect.

And don't be taken in by the popular idea that puffing pot is another harmless pastime. Scientists now feel they have evidence that smoking marijuana may be directly linked with the following: impairment of driving skills, increased sensitivity to pain, a rise in blood pressure with increased heartbeat, headache, tiredness, illusions, feelings of anxiety and alienation, a lack of concentration, birth defects, a weakening of the body's immunity to disease, temporary loss of memory, a loss of appetite, difficulty sleeping, sexual impotency, male sterility, and increased risk of cancer.[12]

Coffee

Let's take a brief look at that innocent-looking cup of coffee. "Wait a minute!" I can hear some of you saying already. "I've known for a long time that cigarettes are a threat to my well-being. I've grudgingly admitted that I'd be better off without my cocktail. I've even told my wife she can hold back on the second piece of my favorite German chocolate cake. But you're really meddling when you begin to cast doubts on my coffee drinking; that's the only thing that keeps me going through the day. In the morning I need a pick-me-up to get rolling, and coffee does the trick. It does the same thing when I have a letdown during the day. If I get jittery, it calms my nerves. On vacation I can drive longer at night without getting sleepy if I have a cup or two of coffee. Let's not knock anything that does so much good."

There's a certain amount of truth in what you say. When you're beginning to feel dragged out, coffee does *seem* to give you a welcome lift. But the problem is, that temporary "shot in the arm" may be costing you more than you suspect.

Let's use a simple example to illustrate what is actually taking place. Say we have a large draft horse capable of pulling heavy wagonloads. Up at the crack of dawn, we put him in harness and begin hauling some unusually heavy loads. Hour after hour he tugs at the collar, and by noon he's ready to be put out to pasture. But we have a lot we want to get done today, so it's more of the same through the long afternoon.

By suppertime, the faithful animal is really exhausted and badly in need of rest. Any more demands on his already weary system will obviously be detrimental to his health. But we have a job we think has to be finished today, so out comes the whip. There aren't any representatives from the Humane Society around, and the poor old horse stumbles along through the dark driven by the relentless lash.

Not a very pretty picture. But when you use coffee for a pick-me-up you're just whipping a "poor old tired horse." True it works, but you are merely borrowing from your energy reserves, and that debt will have to be paid eventually—perhaps with high interest.

The reason coffee seems to have magical lifting powers is because it contains a powerful stimulant called caffeine. This stimulant gives your body a temporary lift, but inevitably this will be followed by a corresponding letdown. That's probably when you reach for the whip again. Let's note what some of the interest payments might be for these unreasonable demands upon your system.

Heart trouble

One study indicates the more coffee you drink the greater your chance of having a heart attack. Those who drink five cups of coffee per day (a rather common intake) have about twice as great a risk of having an acute heart attack as people who do not use coffee at all.[13]

Hypoglycemia and diabetes

Caffeine has an insidious way of blocking some of the body's controlling mechanisms, so that abnormal amounts of sugar are released into the blood stream. Even two cups of coffee can cause a significant rise. This is followed by a corresponding low. Since coffee drinking interferes with the body's sugar regulating system, it also aggravates diabetes.[14]

Digestive problems

Caffeine is only one of the "bad guys" hiding in the coffee bean. Also present are certain oils called "caffeols," which are released when the beans are roasted. These caffeols have a way of irritating those stomach cells that produce acid to help digest food, and consequently these cells get a false message. Although there may be little or no food on hand, they faithfully pour out a nice batch of acid. The end result is one new ulcer patient.

Chromosomes

Chromosomes are extremely important because they are the carriers of hereditary factors from parent to offspring. Caffeine has the ability to damage the chromosomes in human cells.

Nerves

We've already pointed out the pattern of lift and letdown, lift and letdown, so common among coffee users. This continual seesawing effect plays havoc with the body's central nervous system and the results are often irritability, loss of sleep, rapid heartbeat, and muscle tremor. Don't be deceived by the apparent calming effect a cup of coffee momentarily provides.

Tea

And how does tea fit into the picture? Very neatly. A cup of tea contains about the same amount of caffeine as does a cup of coffee, so we should expect about the same effects on the human system. For some reason the results of drinking tea do not seem to parallel the results of coffee drinking as far as heart attack is concerned. Something besides caffeine must be at work in coffee. But otherwise one is about as bad as the other. You won't find your good fortune in your tea leaves.

Anything else?

Don't forget the cola drinks. Their great popularity around the world is not due solely to their admittedly good flavor. A 12-ounce bottle contains more than half as much caffeine as a cup of instant coffee.[15] That's why you'll find so many people crowded around the soda pop machine about the middle of the morning. Like most Americans they have probably skipped breakfast entirely or had a skimpy one at best. Now they are hard at work and the body is running out of steam. A bottle of cola drink will give them that false sense of energy input. The old whip story all over again.

Since true temperance calls for "total abstinence from that which is harmful," obviously anything laced with caffeine is on the no-no list.

Allowing the laws to work for you

We shouldn't leave this subject without pointing out the positive aspects of the matter. Remember that the laws of health are good laws. They cause trouble only when we break them. If we adjust our life-style to be in harmony with them, we can count on a payoff on the plus side of the ledger. Allow me to relate a personal experience showing the truth of this statement.

My father is a dentist; my mother was known as an outstanding cook. Unfortunately we evaluated food only by its effect on the taste buds. Our table groaned with highly refined, fatty foods, and each meal ended with a sugar-laden dessert. This all made for thoroughly epicurean pleasures, but unfortunately conflicted with certain basic health principles. And some of those laws had to do with man's chewing apparatus.

By the time I turned 23, I had become one of my father's

most frequently seen patients. I spent hours in the dental chair, hating every minute of it.

At that point I made two changes in my life-style that for me were to have far-reaching effects. I cut my sugar consumption almost to zero and began brushing my teeth immediately after every meal. (Did you ever think how foolish it is to jump out of bed, brush one's teeth, and then go down to breakfast? One of the main reasons for brushing is to remove food particles.) Was it worth it? *From that time to this, for 29 years, I have never had a single cavity!* Of course, I still have the original gold work, but I also have all of my teeth and my mouth remains in a continual state of perfect health. Somehow I prefer this to the expense of buying dentures, not to mention the joys of trying to learn to use them.

Perhaps I should take a moment to explain why there was such a dramatic turnabout in my dental health. Recent findings seem to indicate two basic reasons. First, dentists now recommend we practice something called "plaque control." Plaque is a sticky, colorless, nearly transparent film, which continuously forms on the teeth. It is made up mostly of bacteria, along with saliva and debris. When ordinary sugars come into contact with certain bacteria found in plaque they immediately form acids. These acids then attack the enamel covering of the teeth leading to the process of decay. Faithful brushing and flossing of the teeth after each meal keeps the surfaces slick, and plaque never has an opportunity to build up! That's what is meant by the term "plaque control."

Ask your dentist about proper brushing and flossing technique. If you can't get to your toothbrush after a meal, at least vigorously rinse your mouth with clean water. And remember that time is of the essence. Most of the damage is done within thirty minutes from the time you finish eating, so don't delay.

Also use care in selecting your toothbrush; again your dentist can advise. Be sure to pick a brush with reasonably soft bristles, because harsh ones can saw right into your tooth enamel.

Recent findings have brought to light even more interesting information. Teeth may appear to be formed out of solid material, but we now know that minute tubes extend from the inside of each tooth right out to the enamel. In a healthy tooth, fluid is constantly moving through these tubes from the inner portion to the outer. If proper nutrients are available in this fluid, and if the rate of flow is rather rapid, all is well. Trouble begins when the rate of fluid flow in the teeth slows down. That is an unhealthy condition that invites dental decay.[16] What can slow down the rate of flow? A heavy sugar intake—in other words the typical American diet. Unless you really enjoy the time you spend in the dental chair, the better part of wisdom is to cut back drastically on sugar consumption. Not only will your teeth benefit, but your entire system, as well. Where health is concerned, sugar is strictly bad news.

So there you have it; cause to effect. The process seems simple enough and yet sometimes we are a little slow to learn.

[1] News Release. Baltimore: The Johns Hopkins Medical Institutions, Nov. 5, 1973.

[2] "Alcoholic Glycemia," British Medical Journal 1:463-4, 1968.

[3] "Fighting Alcoholism," Wall Street Journal, Tuesday, May 23, 1972.

[4] "Alcoholism: New Victims, New Treatments," Reader's Digest, August, 1974, p. 116.

[5] Ibid.

[6] Ibid.

[7] Ibid.

[8] Glenn D. Everett, "Drinking Damages the Brain—Permanently," Listen, December, 1969, pp. 6-8.

[9] Mervyn G. Hardinge, M.D., "Payments Come Due!" Life and Health, March, 1974, pp. 8, 9.

[10] "Does Smoking Really Cause Emphysema?" Life and Health, September, 1972, p. 6.

[11] Mervyn G. Hardinge, M.D., "The Effects of Tobacco Smoke on Nonsmokers," Life and Health, August, 1973, p. 9.

[12] "Cannabis and Driving Skills," C.M.A. Journal, Aug. 19, 1972, pp. 269, 270. See also D. Harvey Powelson, M.D., "Marijuana: More Dangerous Than You Know," Reader's Digest, December, 1974, pp. 95-99.

[13] H. Jick, O. S. Miettinen, R. F. Neff, S. Shapiro, O. P. Heinonon, D. Slone, "Coffee and Myocardial Infarction." A report from the Boston Collaborative Drug Surveillance Program, Boston University Medical Center, New England Journal of Medicine 289:63-67, 1973.

[14] Marjorie V. Baldwin, "Caffeine on Trial," Life and Health, October, 1973, pp. 10-15.

[15] Ibid., p. 12.

[16] Ralph Steinman, D.D.S., "To Brush or Not to Brush," Life and Health, July, 1973, pp. 15-17.

THE
AMBULANCE
OR THE FENCE?

FEAR CLUTCHED our hearts as we heard the news. Bob, the outstanding young high school student who lived just across the hall, had been taken to the hospital. Paralysis had already crept into his neck muscles and soon he was fighting for breath in an iron lung. In a few days the battle was over. The personable teen-ager, the top scholar, the local football star, our friend, was dead.

It was 1953, and a frightening polio epidemic was sweeping across the United States killing scores of youngsters and crippling hundreds of others. Each young person was a potential victim and parents lived in constant fear their home might be the next invaded.

The night after Bob was taken away, we bundled up our little girl and set off for another State. The dreaded disease had touched our own apartment building and we decided it best to leave her with grandparents for a time. Whether this action was valid or not I don't know, but at least we felt we were doing something protective.

How many over the centuries have feared for their lives during mysterious epidemics. Through lack of knowledge, man has been at the mercy of spreading disease. Millions have fallen before the onslaught of bubonic plague, small-

pox, cholera, and typhoid. But one by one these silent killers have been brought largely under control by modern
medical science. The latest news is truly encouraging.

An ancient scourge defeated

A startling announcement early in 1975 declared smallpox soon will be completely wiped out, possibly within a
few months.[1] If so, it will be the first disease to have been
truly eradicated by man.

This devastating illness has ravaged mankind from the
dawn of recorded history. Fifteen years after the discovery
of America, smallpox was introduced into the Western
Hemisphere by the Spaniards, and within a short time 3.5
million of an estimated 6 million natives were said to have
died from it.

During the Middle Ages smallpox was known to have
killed 25 to 30 per cent of the European population in a
single epidemic. As late as 1974 more than 100,000 people
in India were stricken, and an estimated 20,000 died.

But victory appears imminent. The World Health
Organization searches out those suspected of being infected,
then vaccinates everyone within the area while maintaining
a heavy quarantine until the threat is over. The program
has been so successful that only a scattering of a few countries of Asia and Africa still report cases. There have been
no cases of smallpox in the United States for 25 years.

While we hail this good news, the picture is not entirely bright. What we have gained in one area we seem to
have lost in another. Now chronic, degenerative diseases,
particularly those associated with the circulatory and respiratory systems, have become the major source of illness
and death. This is true not only in the United States but in
most affluent countries around the world.

The number one way to go

Perhaps we ought to consider seriously the reason for
our apparent helplessness in the light of advanced medical

knowledge. Where have we gone wrong?

Our most prominent way of dying now is from heart disease. *Atherosclerosis* is a clogging and narrowing of the blood vessels. The blood still has to force its way through the system; it does so under increasing resistance. And eventually the blood supply is completely cut off. If the blood supply to the brain is interrupted the individual suffers a stroke; if a coronary artery supplying the heart muscle is blocked the result is heart attack.

Each year more than a million persons in this country suffer heart attack, and about 700,000 of them die. In fact, heart attack kills one out of every five American men before they reach the age of 60.

Much research is being directed toward this present scourge, and evidence points toward a multiple causation. That is, it appears that several factors combine to produce the disease. Let's look at eight of these factors that profile the person most apt to suffer a heart attack.

1. High blood cholesterol, which may result from the intake of foods high in animal fats.

2. High blood pressure.

3. Cigarette smoking.

4. Physical inactivity.

5. Continuing stress or tension.

6. Obesity.

7. High triglycerides (blood fat), which may result from a liberal use of sugar.

8. An inherited tendency toward the disease.

How do *you* rate on this check list? If none of these apply to you, then you are not a likely candidate for a heart attack. If only one of these factors apply, then you're still in a pretty good position. However, as more of these conditions do apply, one's chances of becoming a premature fatality statistic rise very rapidly.

Is there anything we can do about this number one health problem? This is a most fascinating question. Let's consider these important factors one at a time:

9

1. We can avoid animal fats, and go easy on all saturated fats.

2. Medication can keep blood pressure in line. Food should be salted only lightly.

3. Cigarettes can be given up completely.

4. We can begin a regular exercise program.

5. We can learn to avoid or properly relate to stress or tension.

6. It is possible to bring weight into line and keep it there.

7. The use of table sugar can be kept to a minimum.

8. We can't do much about selecting our parents; that was done for us.

Did you catch the vital point? Out of these eight major factors linked with heart disease, *we can control all but one!* The problem has to do with the way modern man lives. More than better remedies for heart attacks that have already occurred, we need to live in such a way that they never happen at all. We need to develop a proper life-style as early as possible and then stay with it for a lifetime. A longer and better lifetime.

A new way of life

With the progress modern medical science has made, there's no excuse for today's death rate. We're practicing a benign form of suicide; killing ourselves with our soft, luxurious style of living. It's time to quit drifting and to put into actual practice the things we have been talking about in this book. We know what to do; let's do it while there's still opportunity.

A person who honestly wants to take care of himself must understand how the various parts of his body function. The average man knows a lot more about how things work under the hood of his car than he does about his own digestive system. And most women know more about the art of camouflage than they do about keeping their bodies youthful to begin with.

"If the quality of health is to be maintained and improved, we cannot rely on haphazardly acquired information, modern advertising, or the advice of well-meaning friends. Effective decisions imply knowledge. Decisions in matters of health behavior are sound only insofar as they are based on accurate information." [2]

For easy-to-understand help on the make-up of the body and its functions, turn to page 151.

Prevention better than cure

Although illness often seems to come on suddenly, usually it has been developing over a period of time, perhaps years. We are first aware something is wrong when we observe certain symptoms indicating the body is not functioning properly. Even when these signals appear, we often delay doing anything about the problem. Fear of knowing the full truth, or just plain busyness may keep us from acting until the matter is more serious than there was ever any need for it to be. Sometimes we delay until the disease has made irreversible inroads on our system, and nothing can be done except to ease our exit from this life. Symptoms are warnings we cannot afford to ignore.

There is an even safer course to follow. Before the first symptoms of disease appear, the body faithfully produces *signs*. These are evidences of trouble that the victim himself is not aware of, but which can be detected by a physician or dentist. This is why the regular, periodic examination is so important. Many lives could be saved and much discomfort avoided if only people would have an annual checkup. It is one of those onerous little duties so hard to schedule, but the payoff is great in terms of health and happiness. Why not make it a set practice for all the members of your family?

Build a fence

Perhaps some of you remember reading the humorous poem about a village with a problem. Situated near the edge of a cliff, its citizens kept falling over the edge and getting badly hurt. Finally the town council met to remedy the situation once and for all. Unfortunately the council split into two opposing factions, each side loudly championing its own solution.

One group stoutly insisted the logical thing was to purchase an ambulance to stand by at the bottom of the cliff. That way, victims could have immediate attention and be driven quickly to the nearest hospital.

The other camp, equally insistent, felt their money could better be spent in erecting a fence at the edge of the cliff. That way no one would fall off in the first place. The poem is humorous because one approach is so sound and the other so foolish.

Which is to say that, when it comes to health, we've all been tempted to play the fool. Right? We've been "ambulance people," waiting until we're already victims of disease before doing anything constructive.

Our new goal, however, is to adopt a life-style that will keep us in good health and ward off the advances of age. It's time to build that fence.

---

[1] News Release. Health Insurance News, Health Insurance Institute, New York, January, 1975.

[2] John LaPlace, *Health* (New York: Appleton-Century-Crofts, 1972), p. 4.

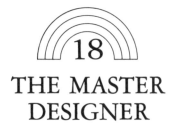

THE MASTER
DESIGNER

YOU'RE NOT going to believe this, but I'm going to tell you anyway. You've probably become somewhat accustomed to the marvels of miniaturization made possible by our advanced space-age technology. But consider a tiny camera no larger than an ordinary ice cube, yet tough enough to last a lifetime. No problem of getting ready to shoot only to find you've forgotten to purchase film for this little wonder. Its single, self-developing, full-color film is capable of recording billions of snapshots. And hold on, this is not merely a still camera but a motion-picture camera capable of handling some 36,000 exposures per hour!

Impossible? Not really. *It's called the human eye.* Strange, isn't it, how many things we tend to take for granted. But let Dr. Irwin Ross tell you more about this fantastic, living camera:

"Light first reaches the eye through a curved window, the cornea. This transparent structure covers the eyeball in front something like the glass of a wrist watch.

"The cornea is cleaned frequently. The upper eyelids act as windshield wipers when you blink, which you do every three seconds or so. Tear glands supply fluid to wash off dust. The fluid even kills germs as it cleans.

"Behind the cornea lies a self-regulating shutter called the iris. Look up at the night sky and pick out the faintest star you can see. The pupil of your eye, the black spot at the center of the colored iris, opens wide to let in as much light as possible. A sunny landscape is some 10 million times brighter. But you still can make out details and distinguish more than 150 hues of the rainbow colors as your pupil contracts to a pinpoint and reduces glare.

"Such adjustments would be impossible without a neatly constructed light meter. Your eyes are hooked up to special nerve centers that measure brightness and automatically set the size of the pupils.

"Like any good seeing instrument, the eye has a light-focusing lens. But nature's version surpasses anything ever manufactured.

"Imagine a plastic as transparent as Lucite, as elastic as rubber, as tough as leather, as efficient as high-grade optical glass and built to last a lifetime. This miracle material makes up the lens of the eye. Attached to strong ligaments, it can be pulled into hundreds of different shapes for near and far vision by the ciliary muscles of the eye.

"The lens also serves as a color filter. Our eyes do not see well by the shortest light waves, which are the colors at the extreme violet end of the visible spectrum. So the eye lens is slightly tinted to filter out such colors. . . .

"The entire apparatus of the eyeball—window, shutter, lens—turns with the aid of six tiny ribbon-shaped muscles that help direct your gaze as accurately as a spotlight beam.

"The cells of the retina perform a host of duties. Some 130 million of these cells are microscopic rods sensitive to low-level illumination. They provide facts about only the general shape and distance of objects and are better for night-time vision.

"For seeing fine details of shapes in *color* under brighter daylight conditions, 7 million cone-shaped cells are used.

An extra-dense population of cones is concentrated within a tiny zone, a barely detectable pit sunk in a yellow-colored shallow depression called the macula. . . . The tiny central pit is called the *fovea* (Latin for 'small pit') *centralis*. It represents the most wonderful of all features of the eye. It makes possible sharp definition of the object in direct view, and involves activities such as sharp focusing for reading small print, examining objects through a microscope, assembling a wrist watch. Under proper conditions you can distinguish between two points much less than one ten-thousandth of an inch apart." [1]

There is more, much more, but perhaps this is sufficient to remind us of the almost unbelievable complexity of the human body. With David, the psalmist, we are led to proclaim, "Thank you for making me so wonderfully complex! It is amazing to think about. Your workmanship is marvelous" (Ps. 139:14, T.L.B.).

No matter what portion of the human body we consider, we find this same pattern of beautifully designed elements working together smoothly to make up the masterpiece that is man. The tiny, delicate bones of the middle ear, the several functions of a hair follicle, the secret inner world of a single cell; all are part of a system so involved that even the greatest minds have yet to fully understand its workings.

It should be obvious to any thinking person that the human form didn't "just happen." Such a marvelous creation testifies to a Creator, a Master Designer. "The hearing ear and the seeing eye, the Lord has made them both" (Prov. 20:12, Revised Standard Version). Man is the handiwork of God.

Instructions are available

You've heard the saying, "If nothing else works, try reading the instructions." Whenever my wife buys a new electrical appliance for the home, I always urge her to read the information sheet before plugging it in and flipping the switch. The company that manufactured the product knows precisely how it operates and what precautions should be taken. In case of malfunction, helpful suggestions are usually included.

It stands to reason that the One who created man in the beginning knows most about him and how he best functions. Fortunately He has also provided an instruction book— the Holy Bible. In it a servant of God states: "I pray that all may go well with you and that you may be in health" (3 John 2, Revised Standard Version).

The question immediately comes to mind, "If that truly reflects God's desire for His creation, then why is there so much illness in the world?" It's apparent that an antagonistic force is also at work, a power opposed to all that is good. We need to be careful about referring to various calamaties as "acts of God." That may serve as a legal term, but it certainly isn't accurate. God's desire is always that we "be in health."

Earlier in this book we talked about the wonder of healing in a wound. The attending physician realizes he has very little to do with the miracle of restoration that takes place. A power far greater than his own is in evidence. The Bible points to the source of that power; "I am the Lord, your healer" (Ex. 15:26, Revised Standard Version).

One of the many titles attributed to Christ is "the Great Physician." According to Holy Writ, it would appear Christ actually spent more time healing than He did preaching. His voice was the first many ever heard, His name the first they ever spoke, His face the first they ever gazed upon. With infinite compassion He made His way through the dusty by-ways of Palestine, bringing healing and hope to all.

An ancient book on health

We would expect the Bible to have some helpful suggestions in regard to health. But is it possible for such an ancient document to contain information still relevant and reliable for our own day? The answer, surprisingly, is Yes.

Let's note a few specific examples.

During the Middle Ages devastating plagues took the lives of millions upon millions of people. This frightening loss of life could have been avoided, and finally was brought under control, by implementing techniques for dealing with contagious diseases as outlined in Leviticus 13.[2]

Up until the close of the eighteenth century even the great cities of the world had virtually no hygienic provisions. Excrement was simply dumped into the streets; flies multiplied, resulting in the spread of disease. More millions of lives were lost. Even with the lack of technical knowledge in those days, large scale loss of life could have been avoided by following the simple precautions outlined in Deuteronomy 23.

As late as the nineteenth century large numbers of mothers died from infections following childbirth because physicians attended them just after doing autopsies. Disease was carried from the dead to the living. This need not have been the case had the admonition in Numbers 19 been followed; hands should be carefully washed in running water after touching a dead body.

Adherence to the Bible prohibition against eating swine's flesh would have kept people from contracting trichinosis. Fortunately the incidence of this disease in America today is lessening, but in the thirties and forties some 16 per cent of our total population was infected.[3]

Nature's laws

Earlier we talked about nature's unchanging laws, and pointed out that disease comes from either ignorantly or willfully violating those laws of health. It's a simple matter of cause and effect:

Cause		Effect
Disobedience	=	Disease
Obedience	=	Health

It is important to understand that nature's laws are di-

vinely ordained. God is the author of both moral and physical law. They have been written by His own finger upon
every nerve, every muscle, every faculty entrusted to man.
Never should the rules of health be taken lightly, as though
they were of little consequence.

Man and his spirit

We have considered the physical and mental aspects of
man, and how they sympathize one with the other. It is
vital to recognize that man is actually a three-dimensional
creature, with a moral or spiritual nature, as well. Man is
body and mind and spirit. If man is truly to be made
whole, then we must deal with the whole man.

The average person takes much better care of his automobile than he does his own body. This is rather strange
when we consider it is possible to purchase another car,
while the body we receive at birth has to last a lifetime.
Because of abuse or neglect, that "lifetime" is too often
relatively brief. Our bodies simply give up and cease to
function.

Some consider the body not only of little consequence
but even something to be mistreated. I personally have
witnessed so-called "holy men" abusing themselves in pa-
thetic ways. Sincere, but sincerely mistaken.

Others take the attitude that what they do with their
bodies is no one else's business. Wrong again. The truth is
we *are* accountable for the manner in which we take care,
or do not take care, of ourselves:

"Haven't you yet learned that your body is the home of
the Holy Spirit God gave you, and that he lives within
you? Your own body does not belong to you. For God has
bought you with a great price. So use every part of your
body to give glory back to God, because he owns it" (1
Cor. 6:19, 20, T.L.B.).

We did not create ourselves. Birth is merely a continu-
ation of that Edenic miracle when God brought into existence the first man. "Then the Lord God formed man of

dust from the ground, and breathed into his nostrils the breath of life; and man became a living being" (Gen. 2:7, Revised Standard Version).

Whether we confess it or not, we are individually the property of God. It is He who has formed us; we are His by right of creation.

But God has a double claim upon us. We are His not only because He created us but also because He redeemed us at great cost. "For God loved the world so much that he gave his only Son so that everyone who believes in him should not be lost, but should have eternal life" (John 3:16, Phillips).[4]

It does make a difference how we care for ourselves. We are accountable for our life-style and its effects on body, mind, and spirit.

When man came forth from the hand of the Creator he was perfect in every respect. Millenniums of degeneration have left us poor copies of the original design. Our solemn responsibility is to cooperate with God in a great work of restoration. As Adam was created in the image of God, so we once again should reflect His goodness in body, mind, and spirit.

---

[1] Irwin Ross, Ph.D., "Nature's Marvelous Camera," *Life and Health*, March, 1973, pp. 18-20.

[2] George Rosen, *History of Public Health* (New York: MD Publications, 1958), pp. 63-65.

[3] *Trichinosis Surveillance, Annual Summary*, 1968 (Atlanta, Georgia: National Center for Disease Control), May, 1969.

[4] The Bible texts in this book credited to Phillips are from *The New Testament in Modern English*, © J. B. Phillips, 1958. Used by permission of The Macmillan Company.

19

THE ABUNDANT
LIFE

AS THE onions rolled across the pale-blue carpet, guests stared in disbelief. Conversation was halted in midstream, and all eyes turned to the hostess. Her lovely home, meticulously kept, had been under assault now for almost an hour. The time of crisis had arrived.

One of the couples had brought along their nearly-5-year-old son and their 3-year-old daughter. While the mother and father visited in a most relaxed manner, the children were left to explore the house at will. They finally settled on the kitchen as the room with the most potential. As fearful bangings and clankings were heard coming from that direction the hostess looked nervous and apprehensive, but being a sensitive person she held her peace. Now the dynamic duo marched into the living room with a sack of onions and proceeded to dump them unceremoniously in the middle of the room. Then they looked around in satisfaction as though they expected to be warmly applauded for such a performance.

At last the lady of the house decided it might not be out of the way to protect her property as long as she acted gently. But as she rose out of her chair she was motioned back by the mother of the two onion rollers. "Please don't bother them," the latter half whispered. "We're trying to raise them the modern way, without negatives. We don't want to damage their psyche. When they're through playing with the onions, I'll be happy to pick them up."

Checkmated, the hostess sank back into her chair. But one of the male guests was from the old school. His right hand was itching to make direct contact with the dynamic duo, and it was not their psyches he had in mind. Restraining himself with difficulty, he asked bluntly, "What would you do if they brought a saw up from the basement and proceeded to saw a leg off the grand piano?"

Without hesitation the mother replied, "I'd buy our hostess a new piano." And she meant it.

I've often wondered where those youngsters are now and how they are faring. How did they react when they learned, as they must have eventually, that the world outside the home has rules and regulations that have to be observed. That there is a police force to back up civil authority. Did the girl's—now a young woman—mental processes finally break down? Is the young man locked up in some maximum security prison? Or have they learned to adjust to the rest of society in spite of their parents? I hope they have, but if so I'm certain it was only after much bitter relearning in the proverbial school of hard knocks.

Short-circuiting the conscience

For years we have been seeking an easy, nonrestrictive route to happiness and contentment. For the youngsters there has been "permissiveness"; for the adults, "situation ethics." But the formula still eludes us. The greater share of the hospital beds in this country are still filled with people suffering from mental illness, and, I believe, there is less happiness today than before.

Certainly this is the case with many of today's teenagers. When I was growing up we could have a million dollars worth of fun with twenty cents and an old jalopy. Now the younger set is so completely sated with life's "goodies" they don't know what do with themselves. Seeking instant satisfaction, they rush from one piece of action to another—and end up with a chronic case of boredom. This very boredom is one of the roots of violence.

And a new element of fear is abroad in the land. Before we admit guests they must submit to a careful screening through the one-way peephole, and then wait while we undo the triple locks on the door.

There is also growing fear about job security. The national economy teeters on the brink, and somehow we have a feeling things may never be quite the same again.

So why not live a little—or a lot? Turn up the volume, lift the glass, put those restrictive morals away in mothballs. Revel in our newfound "freedom." But down inside we're not even fooling ourselves, let alone others.

Our innate sense of what is right and wrong can't be turned off quite so easily. That deep-seated feeling of guilt is ever with us. And guilt gnaws away at our vitals. It undermines our health and leaves us unsatisfied and unhappy.

Is there an answer to our predicament? The noted psychiatrist Dr. Karl Menninger asks a most intriguing question in the title of his latest book, *What Ever Became of Sin?* This is the kind of question we might expect of a minister, but the pulpit has been evading the issue. Even preachers have been busy staking out a broad, easy route to the kingdom.

Psychologists have been doing some thinking, too. Henry C. Link says, "The emphasis on sin has largely disappeared from the teachings of religion . . . at the very time when psychology has discovered its importance and extended its meaning." [1]

Dr. Menninger feels it is time to once again call sin by its right name. His straightforward admonition to the clergy is, "Preach! Tell it like it is. Say it from the pulpit. Cry it from the housetops. What shall we cry? Cry comfort, cry repentance, cry hope." [2]

The universal quest

As I have traveled around the world I find that people of all lands, irrespective of their differing cultures, are looking for the same thing. It is not a search for wealth, power, or recognition, but for *peace of mind*. All of man's striving, usually futile, is ultimately directed toward this one goal.

That the Christian is engaged in such a quest is strange, for peace of mind is his rightful legacy. Jesus has promised: "Peace is my parting gift to you, my own peace, such as the world cannot give. Set your troubled hearts at rest, and banish your fears" (John 14:27, N.E.B.). [3]

If such peace is our legacy, then how has it evaded us? We have tried desperately to eradicate our guilt feelings by downgrading the codes or rules we were ordained to live by. It hasn't worked. We need instead to do away with our burden of guilt by coming into harmony with heaven's code of conduct, and acquainting ourselves with the divine Author of those commandments.

Harmony and happiness

Remember in chapter two we were trying to define health? Here is yet another characteristic of health to consider: *Good health can be anticipated when one has a harmonious relationship between body, mind, and spirit.* Paul's advice in Romans 14:19 is to the point: "Let us concentrate on the things which make for harmony" (Phillips).

Harmony is happiness, and happiness promotes good health. "A cheerful heart does good like medicine" (Prov. 17:22, T.L.B.).

A consciousness of right-doing is the best medicine for body and mind. Another psychiatrist, Dr. William Sadler, testifies to this fact:

"No one can appreciate so fully as a doctor the amazingly large percentage of human disease and suffering which is directly traceable to worry, fear, conflict, immorality, dissipation, and ignorance—to unwholesome thinking and unclean living. The sincere acceptance of the principles and teachings of Christ with respect to the life of mental peace and joy, the life of unselfish thought and clean living, would at once wipe out more than half the difficulties, diseases, and sorrows of the human race. In other words, more than one half of the present affliction of mankind could be prevented by the tremendous prophylactic power of actually living up to the personal and practical spirit of the real teachings of Christ.

"The teachings of Jesus applied to our modern civilization—understandingly applied, not merely nominally accepted—would so purify, uplift, and vitalize us that the race would immediately stand out as a new order of beings, possessing superior mental power and increased moral force. Irrespective of the future rewards of living, laying aside all discussion of future life, *it would pay any man or woman to live the Christ-life just for the mental and moral rewards it affords here in this present world.* Some day man may awake to the fact that the teachings of Christ are potent and powerful in preventing and curing disease. Some day our boasted scientific development, as regards mental and moral improvement, may indeed catch up with the teachings of this man of Galilee." [4]

A strong statement, indeed, but Dr. Sadler has support in his thesis that a man in tune with the Infinite is a man who will likely enjoy good health. Researchers at Johns Hopkins University have found that churchgoers have fewer illnesses than nonchurchgoers.[5] Drs. Friedman and Rosenman in their book *Type A Behavior and Your Heart* have noted:

"We can declare, however, with considerable certainty, that we have rarely encountered this behavior pattern (the one predisposing to heart attack) in any person whose religious and patriotic beliefs take precedence over his preoccupation with the accumulation of 'numbers' or the acquisition of personal power." [6]

You will recall the strong assumption on the part of

some researchers that stress lies at the root of all disease. The devoutly religious person finds that his personal faith is a great allayer of stress. One reason life has become so stressful in recent years is that many have relegated religion to a minor role or abandoned it altogether. Now, however, people seem to be turning once again to religious faith, particularly of the evangelical type.

What we have proposed in this present book is nothing less than a comprehensive life-style, probably a new one to most readers. To embrace it would likely mean making a number of changes, some of them not easy ones. Old habits would have to be discarded and new ones established. Could it actually be worth it all? Has any group of people tested it out for true effectiveness?

Fortunately, yes. There is a group of people, members of the Seventh-day Adventist Church, who have tried to live in accordance with the health philosophy presented in this volume. They have not always lived up to these high standards in every respect, but generally they have been faithful to these principles. A temperate people, they do not drink or smoke, and largely follow a vegetarian regimen. They take their religion seriously, and consider good health to be an important part of the Christian's way of life.

Some years ago Dr. Frank Lemon (currently associate dean for extramural affairs of the Medical College of the University of Kentucky) and his associates studied the question of health and religion. In comparing Seventh-day Adventists with the general population, they reported the following findings:

"The death risk in this group (SDA's) for respiratory tract disease is very low, and is substantially reduced for other causes of death prevalent in the United States today, such as stroke, coronary heart disease, arteriosclerosis, liver cirrhosis, and cancer. . . .

"We have found that observed deaths among SDA men were about 50 per cent of expected, and among SDA women about 60 per cent of expected." [7]

To put it in even plainer language, *Seventh-day Adventist men live up to six and one-half years longer than the average man!* Not an insignificant portion of a life-span. A real payoff. And yet nothing mysterious; nothing that isn't available to anyone willing to live in harmony with the laws of health.

Who, me?

"This all sounds very wonderful," you may say, "but you don't know me. My intentions are great, but when it comes to the actual doing I'm all marshmallow; no backbone at all. My bad habits are so ingrained I don't think I can ever break loose from some of them."

Courage. You're not the first person who ever felt that way. We think of the apostle Paul as a tough old Christian warrior, but listen to his own personal testimony: "My own behavior baffles me. . . . I often find that I have the will to do good, but not the power. That is, I don't accomplish the good I set out to do, and the evil I don't really want to do I find I am always doing. Yet if I do things that I don't really want to do then it is not, I repeat, "I" who do them, but the sin which has made its home within me. When I come up against the Law I want to do good, but in practice I do evil. My conscious mind wholeheartedly endorses the Law, yet I observe an entirely different principle at work in my nature. This is in continual conflict with my conscious attitude, and makes me an unwilling prisoner to the law of sin and death. In my mind I am God's willing servant, but in my own nature I am bound fast, as I say, to the law of sin and death. It is an agonizing situation, and who on earth can set me free from the clutches of my own sinful nature?" (Rom. 7:15-24, Phillips).

Sound familiar? Your problem isn't really unique at all, is it? Paul experienced the same frustrations you have had to put up with.

With Paul you have probably said also, "Who on earth can set me free?" The answer is, frankly, no one. No one on this earth can give you the resolve to do all the things you know you should do and want to do. Other people are facing exactly the same problem and can offer nothing but sympathy—and you need something a lot stronger than sympathy. But the case isn't hopeless.

Paul found an answer to his problem. The very next verse, verse 25, reads: "I thank God there is a way out through Jesus Christ our Lord."

No one on earth is able to set you free, but Christ can strengthen your resolve. He has faced every temptation you will ever have to face, and done so victoriously. "All power" has been given unto Him, and He stands ready to share that power with you. This is why Paul said later: "I can do everything God asks me to with the help of Christ who gives me the strength and power" (Phil. 4:13, T.L.B.).

"Everything." Nothing is impossible for the one who puts his full confidence in the Lord and lives in harmony with His commandments. We are not speaking of theory, but of fact.

Let me give you a concrete example. Records of stop-smoking clinics indicate those participants with strong religious motivation have an unusually high success rate. My own personal experience bears this out. When I decided to give up smoking nearly thirty years ago, there were no stop-smoking clinics to give assistance. A person was really on his own. I went through the old familiar pattern of stopping again and again, with my good intentions lasting for only a day or so at a stretch. It seemed an impossible challenge. Then I became a Christian and felt I had a right to claim the promise of divine help. With an entirely new motivation I laid aside my cigarette pack, never to pick it up again. I don't feel like much of a hero, because there really wasn't any struggle. The power came entirely from outside.

In his excellent book *None of These Diseases*, Dr. S. I. McMillen tells of two psychiatrists, Dr. William Sadler and his wife, Lena, who were trying to free a patient from a very serious situation. The "refined, highly educated" woman was not responding to even their combined psychiatric counseling. Finally Dr. Sadler advised his wife that she need not expect any worthwhile improvement, "until her patient's mental life was set in order and numerous psychic slivers were removed." When his wife asked how long that might take, he replied, "Probably a year or more." Now let Dr. William Sadler tell you in his own words what happened:

"Imagine my surprise when this patient walked into my office a few days later and informed me that her 'troubles were all over,' that the things she had assured me a few days previously she 'could never do,' had all been done, that everything I had asked her to do as part of her 'cure' had been set in operation—she had completely overhauled her social, family, and personal life, had made numerous 'confessions,' and had accomplished a score of almost impossible mental and 'moral' stunts.

"In reply to my astonished question, 'How in the world did you ever do all this and effect this great change in your mental attitude toward yourself and the world in less than one week?' she smilingly replied, 'Dr. Lena taught me to pray!' " [8]

Although prayer may seem mysterious to some, it is simply opening up one's heart to God as to a friend. It is an intimate conversation with the Divine, from whom all strength and goodness derives. Strange that more of us do not take advantage of this most precious opportunity.

Many physicians will admit they have seen patients respond to prayer for healing in a manner that defies all natural law. The eminent Dr. Alexis Carrel in his book *Prayer Is Power* wrote: "Prayer is a force as real as terrestrial gravity. As a physician, I have seen men, after all other therapy had failed, lifted out of disease and melancholy by the serene effort of prayer. It is the only power in the world that seems to overcome the so-called 'laws of nature;' the occasions on which prayer has dramatically done this have been termed 'miracles.' But a constant, quieter miracle takes place hourly in the hearts of men and women who have discovered that prayer supplies them with a steady flow of sustaining power in their daily lives."

Designed to live

Along with me, you probably have had a suspicion that many manufactured items could be made to last much longer than they do—and probably at the same cost. The fine art of designing things so they break down after a set number of hours of operation is perhaps necessary to our type of economy; I don't know. But, anyway, that is not the way God designed man.

Each cell of the body is fantastically complex, and the whole human system operates with such perfect harmony as to be almost beyond comprehension. The greatest minds in the world have yet to master its innermost secrets. Surely it should be apparent that man was designed to live longer than the brief "three score years and ten." Let's take another look at a favorite Bible quotation: "For God loved the world so much that he gave his only Son so that everyone who believes in him should not be lost, but should have eternal life" (John 3:16, Phillips).

Not just a few brief years of trial and trouble in this old world, but eternal life without trials and trouble. A life without fear, pain, sickness, or death. This is the hope that Christ holds out to us, and He is capable of providing it.

Is this a lottery? Something for the fortunate few? No, God says, "everyone." That means me, and it means you. Life without end is within the grasp of every believing man and woman. A gift provided at infinite cost, but lovingly offered to us without price.

If you have never known Christ as a personal Friend, but would like to enter into a new relationship with Him, you will want to accept the offer on page 159.

And remember, we are speaking not only of the future,

we are also talking of the here and now. It is in this present world that we are to begin our enjoyment of things eternal. "And what is it that God has said? That he has given us eternal life, and that this life is in his Son. So whoever has God's Son has life; whoever does not have his Son, does not have life" (1 John 5:11,12, T.L.B.).

Notice the present tense, *"has* life." God is the very source of all life, and when we are linked with Him we have this life within ourselves. As long as we choose to remain in close relationship with Him, we have nothing to fear even in this present world.

Christ came not to restrict our freedoms as many suppose, but to introduce us to a richer, fuller life in Him. He says, "I have come that men may have life, and may have it in all its fullness" (John 10:10, N.E.B.). The abundant life is what we are advocating. The entire man, completely whole in body, mind, and spirit. Should we settle for less? All can be ours.

---

[1] Henry C. Link, *The Way to Security* (Garden City, New York: Doubleday and Company, Inc., 1951), p. 52.

[2] Karl Menninger, M.D., *Whatever Became of Sin?* (New York: Hawthorne Books, Inc., 1973), p. 228.

[3] Texts credited to N.E.B. are from *The New English Bible.* © The Delegates of the Oxford University Press and the Syndics of the Cambridge University Press, 1970. Reprinted by permission.

[4] William Sadler, M.D., *Practice of Psychiatry* (St. Louis: C. V. Mosby Company, 1953), p. 1,008.

[5] G. W. Comstock, K. B. Partridge, "Church Attendance and Health," *Journal of Chronic Diseases* 25:665-673. 1972.

[6] Meyer Friedman, M.D., Ray Rosenman, M.D., *Type A Behavior and Your Heart* (New York: Alfred A. Knopf, 1974), p. 169.

[7] F. R. Lemon, J. W. Kuzma, "A Biological Cost of Smoking," *Arch. of Environmental Health*, 19:950-955 (June) 1969.

[8] William Sadler, *Theory and Practice of Psychiatry* (St. Louis: C. V. Mosby Co., 1936), p. 1,075.

APPENDIX

Note: Prices are subject to change.

Health Journals

Life and Health. A monthly family magazine featuring up-to-date, scientifically accurate, health information. Written for laymen in a clear, easy-to-read style. $8.00 per year.

Obesity (a *Life and Health* Supplement). A comprehensive treatment of an important problem. $2.00 each.

Vegetarianism (a *Life and Health* Supplement). Beautifully illustrated booklet covering all aspects of vegetarianism. $1.50 each.

For any of the above, write to:
Life and Health
Review and Herald Publishing Association
6856 Eastern Avenue NW.
Washington, D.C. 20012

Listen. A monthly journal of better living, providing a vigorous, positive educational approach to the problems arising out of the use of tobacco, alcohol, and narcotics. $6.50 per year. Write to a book center listed on page 154 or:
Listen
Pacific Press Publishing Association
1350 Villa Street
Mountain View, California 94042

Health Books

The Miracle of Life	$ .65
The Wonderful Human Machine (English)	.50
(Spanish)	2.60

Order Department
American Medical Association
535 North Dearborn Street
Chicago, Illinois 60610

Other health books are available from book centers listed on page 154.

Health Assistance Programs

Write for information as to when the following programs will be offered in your area:

Five-Day Plan to Stop Smoking
Four-Dimensional Key to Better Living Without Alcohol or Drugs
Home Nursing and First-Aid Classes
Nutrition and Cooking School
Wā-Rite Weight Management Program

Address for any of above programs:

6840 Eastern Avenue NW.
Washington, D.C. 20012

Health Courses

Your World of Good Health	$1.00
Your World of Good Food	1.00

P.O. Box 3838
Hollywood, California 90028

Living for Real   No Charge

Box 100
Thousand Oaks, California 91360

Recipe Books

Order from book center nearest your home as listed on page 154 or from the following address:

ABC Mailing Service
2621 Farnham Street
Omaha, Nebraska 68131

Adventures in Vegetarian Cooking, spiral bound	$3.95
An Apple a Day, spiral bound	4.95
Better Meals for Less, soft cover	1.50
Century 21 Cookbook, spiral bound (English and Spanish)	3.00
Dining Delightfully, spiral bound	4.95
Good Foods for Good Health, spiral bound	4.95
Oats, Peas, Beans, and Barley Cookbook, soft cover	4.50
Vegetarian Cookery Set (Five Volumes), spiral bound	9.95

Religious Journals

The following religious magazines minister to the whole man—body, mind, and spirit.

These Times (Monthly) $8.00 per year

Circulation Department
Southern Publishing Association
Box 59
Nashville, Tennessee 37202

Signs of the Times (Monthly)   8.00 per year

Circulation Department
Pacific Press Publishing Association
1350 Villa Street
Mountain View, California 94042

Message Magazine (Bi-monthly)   5.00 per year

Circulation Department
Southern Publishing Association
Box 59
Nashville, Tennessee 37202

The Ministry (A journal for ministers)   8.95 per year

Circulation Department
Review and Herald Publishing Association
6856 Eastern Avenue NW.
Washington, D.C. 20012

Religious Books

A wide variety of religious books may be obtained from book centers listed on page 154.

Vegetarian Foods

A wide variety of canned and frozen vegetable-protein foods is available at many of the following centers:

Book Centers

The following centers serve as distribution points for journals, books, and vegetarian foods. Write the one nearest you.

UNITED STATES

Alabama-Mississippi Book Center
6650 Atlanta Highway
Box 3508
Montgomery, Alabama 36109

Alaska Book Center
718 Barrow Street
Anchorage, Alaska 99501

Allegheny East Book Center
1287 Penn Avenue
Reading, Pennsylvania 19610

Allegheny West Book Center
Fairgrounds & Wooster Rds.
P.O. Box 831
Mt. Vernon, Ohio 43050

Arizona Book Center
320 North 44th Street
(P.O. Box 21147) (85036)
Phoenix, Arizona 85008

Arkansas-Louisiana Book Center
339 Southfield Road
(P.O. Box 5548)
Shreveport, Louisiana 71105

Carolina Book Center
6000 Conference Dr.
Box 25848
Charlotte, North Carolina 28212

Central California Book Center
1691 The Alamode
(P.O. Box 580) (95106)
San Jose, California 95106

Central States Book Center
5737 Swope Parkway
(P.O. Box 1527) (64141)
Kansas City, Missouri 64130

Chesapeake Book Center
1201 Columbia Pike, Box 803
Columbia, Maryland 21043

Colorado Book Center
2520 South Downing
Denver, Colorado 80210

Florida Book Center
2420 Camden Road
(P.O. Box 1313) (32802)
Orlando, Florida 32803

Georgia-Cumberland Book Center
P.O. Box 4929
Atlanta, Georgia 30302

Greater New York Book Center
227 West Forty-sixth Street
New York, New York 10036

Hawaiian Book Center
2728 Pali Highway
(P.O. Box 4037) (96813)
Honolulu, Hawaii 96813

Idaho Book Center
7777 Fairview
Boise, Idaho 83704

Illinois Book Center
3725 Prairie Avenue
(P.O. Box 29)
Brookfield, Illinois 60513

Indiana Book Center
1405 Broad Ripple Avenue
Indianapolis, Indiana 46220

Iowa Book Center
1200 Twelfth Street
(P.O. Box 475)
West Des Moines, Iowa 50265

Kansas Book Center
3330 Urish Road
(P.O. Box 4526) (66604)
Topeka, Kansas 66614

Kentucky-Tennessee Book Center
600 Hospital Road
(P.O. Box 1277,
Madison College Branch)
Madison, Tennessee 37115

Lake Region Book Center
3725 Prairie Ave.
P.O. Box 29
Brookfield, Illinois 60513

Michigan Book Center
320 West St. Joseph Street
(P.O. Box 900) (48904)
Lansing, Michigan 48933

Minnesota Book Center
1100 Ford Road at Hwy. 12
Minnetonka, Minnesota 55343

Missouri Book Center
8540 Blue Ridge Boulevard
(P.O. Box 11540)
Kansas City, Missouri 64138

Montana Book Center
1425 West Main Street
(P.O. Box 743)
Bozeman, Montana 59715

Nebraska Book Center
4745 Prescott Avenue
(P.O. Box 6037)
Lincoln, Nebraska 68506

Nevada-Utah Book Center
1095 East Taylor Street
(P.O. Box 1470)
Reno, Nevada 89505

New Jersey Book Center
2160 Brunswick Avenue
Trenton, New Jersey 08638

New York Book Center
4930 West Seneca Turnpike
(P.O. Box 67)
Syracuse, New York 13215

North Dakota Book Center
1315 Fourth Street NE.
(P.O. Box 1491)
Jamestown, North Dakota 58401

Northeastern Book Center
560 West 150th Street
New York, New York 10031

Northern California Book Center
2300 Norse Drive
(P.O. Box 23165)
Pleasant Hill, California 94523

Northern New England Book
   Center
91 Allen Avenue
(P.O. Box 1340) (04104)
Portland, Maine 04103

Ohio Book Center
Fairground and Wooster Roads
(P.O. Box 831)
Mount Vernon, Ohio 43050

Oklahoma Book Center
Box 32188
4735 NW. 63rd Street
Oklahoma City, Oklahoma 73132

Oregon Book Center
605 SE. Thirty-ninth Avenue
Portland, Oregon 97214

Pennsylvania Book Center
1287 Penn Avenue
Reading, Pennsylvania 19610

Potomac Book Center
8400 Carroll Avenue
Takoma Park, Maryland 20012

South Atlantic Book Center
Box 92447, Morris Brown Sta.
Atlanta, Georgia 30314

South Central Book Center
715 Young's Lane
(P.O. Box 936) (37202)
Nashville, Tennessee 37207

South Dakota Book Center
217 North Grand
(P.O. Box 520)
Pierre, South Dakota 57501

Southeastern California Book
  Center
9707 Magnolia Avenue
(P.O. Box 7584)
Riverside, California 92503

Southern California Book Center
1535 East Chevy Chase Drive
(P.O. Box 969) (91209)
Glendale, California 91206

Southern New England Book
  Center
34 Sawyer Street (Box 848)
South Lancaster, Massachusetts
  01561

Texas Book Center
P.O. Box 686
Keene, Texas 76059

Texico Book Center
P.O. Box 1399
Amarillo, Texas 79105

Upper Columbia Book Center
West 1025 Indiana Avenue
Spokane, Washington 99205

Washington Book Center
1101 N. Allen Place
(P.O. Box 30026)
Seattle, Washington 98103

West Virginia Book Center
1400 Liberty Street
Parkersburg, West Virginia
  26101

Wisconsin Book Center
802 East Gorham Street
(P.O. Box 512) (53701)
Madison, Wisconsin 53703

Wyoming Book Center
3925 Casper Mountain Road
(P.O. Box 620)
Casper, Wyoming 82601

CANADA

Eastern Canada Book Center
1110 King Street, East
P.O. Box 520
Oshawa, Ontario L1H 7M1

Western Canada Book Center
4826 11th Street, NE. Bay 12
Calgary, Alberta
Canada T2E 2W7

BERMUDA

Bermuda Book Center
P.O. Box 1170
Hamilton, Bermuda

Hospitals

The following medical institutions embrace the health philosophy presented in this book:

Ardmore Adventist Hospital
1012—14th Street NW.
Ardmore, Oklahoma 73401

Battle Creek Sanitarium Hospital
197 North Washington Avenue
Battle Creek, Michigan 49016

Boulder Memorial Hospital
311 Mapleton Avenue
Boulder, Colorado 80302

Castle Memorial Hospital
640 Ulukahiki Street
Kailua, Hawaii 96734

Feather River Hospital
5974 Pentz Road
Paradise, California 95969

Florida Hospital
601 E. Rollins Street
Orlando, Florida 32803

Fuller Memorial Hospital
231 Washington Street
South Attleboro, Massachusetts
  02703

Glendale Adventist Medical
  Center
1509 Wilson Terrace
Glendale, California 91206

Hackettstown Community
  Hospital
651 Willow Grove Street
Hackettstown, New Jersey 07840

Hadley Memorial Hospital
4601 Martin Luther King, Jr.
  Ave., SW.
Washington, D.C. 20032

Hanford Community Hospital
P.O. Box 121
Hanford, California 93230

Hays Memorial Hospital
P.O. Box 767
San Marcos, Texas 78666

Highland Hospital
Route 4
Portland, Tennessee 37148

Hinsdale Sanitarium & Hospital
120 North Oak Street
Hinsdale, Illinois 60521

Huguley Memorial SDA Medical
  Center
P.O. Box 1013
Keene, Texas 76059

Jay Memorial Hospital of SDA
Box H
Jay, Oklahoma 74346

Jellico Community Hospital
P.O. Box 118
Jellico, Tennessee 37762

Kettering Medical Center
3535 Southern Boulevard
Kettering, Ohio 45429

Loma Linda University Medical
  Center
11234 Anderson Street
Loma Linda, California 92354

Louis Smith Memorial Hospital
Box 306
Lakeland, Georgia 31635

Madison Hospital
500 Hospital Drive
Madison, Tennessee 37115

Marion County Hospital
P.O. Box 548
Jefferson, Texas 75657

Medical Center Hospital
809 East Marion Avenue
Punta Gorda, Florida 33950

Memorial Hospital
P.O. Box 880
Beeville, Texas 78102

Memorial Hospital, Inc.
401 Memorial Drive
Manchester, Kentucky 40962

Menard Hospital
P.O. Box 608
Menard, Texas 76859

Monument Valley SDA Hospital
P.O. Box 6
Monument Valley, Utah 84536

New England Memorial Hospital
5 Woodland Road
Stoneham, Massachusetts 02180

North York Branson Hospital
555 Finch Avenue, West
Willowdale, Ontario M2R 1N5

Paradise Valley Hospital
2400 East Fourth Street
National City, California 92050

Parkview Memorial Hospital
Mere Point Road
Brunswick, Maine 04011

Porter Memorial Hospital
2525 South Downing Street
Denver, Colorado 80210

Port Hueneme Adventist Hospital
307 East Clara Street
Port Hueneme, California 93041

Portland Adventist Hospital
6040 SE. Belmont Street
Portland, Oregon 97215

Reading Institute of
   Rehabilitation
Route 1, Box 250
Reading, Pennsylvania 19607

Rest Haven General Hospital
10461 Resthaven Drive
Sidney, British Columbia,
   V8L 3R7

Riverside Hospital
800 Youngs Lane
Nashville, Tennessee 37207

St. Helena Hospital & Health
   Center
Deer Park, California 94576

Shawnee Mission Medical Center
74th and Grandview
Shawnee Mission, Kansas 66201

Simi Valley Adventist Hospital
P.O. Box 456
Simi Valley, California 93065

Sonora Community Hospital
1, South Forest Road
Sonora, California 95370

Takoma Hospital
401 Takoma Avenue
Greeneville, Tennessee 37743

Tempe Community Hospital
1500 South Mill Avenue
Tempe, Arizona 85281

Tillamook County General
   Hospital
1000 Third Street
Tillamook, Oregon 97141

Toole County Adventist Hospital
   and Nursing Home
112 First Street South
Shelby, Montana 59474

Walker Memorial Hospital
P.O. Box A
Avon Park, Florida 33825

Walla Walla General Hospital
933 Bonsella
Walla Walla, Washington 99362

Washington Adventist Hospital
7600 Carroll Avenue
Takoma Park, Maryland 20012

Watkins Memorial Hospital
P.O. Box 346
Ellijay, Georgia 30540

White Memorial Medical Center
1720 Brooklyn Avenue
Los Angeles, California 90033

A SPECIAL OFFER

The book *Steps to Christ* is one of the most widely read religious volumes other than the Bible. More than 18 million copies have been printed in 100 different languages. For a complimentary copy of this most helpful and inspiring book, please clip and mail the coupon below:

COME ALIVE! OFFER

cut out and mail to
Review and Herald Publishing Association
6856 Eastern Avenue NW.
Washington, D.C. 20012

Please send a free copy of the book *Steps to Christ* to:

Name ....

Address ....

City .... State .... Zip ....